W9-AZX-312

Rite Aid
# GUIDE TO HEALTH

# Alzheimer's

*Reliable Information for Patients
and Their Families*

CAROLYN DEAN, M.D.

Published by
Adams Media, an F+W Publications Company
57 Littlefield Street
Avon, MA 02322
*www.adamsmedia.com*

ISBN 10: 1-59337-696-0
ISBN 13: 978-1-59337-696-3

Printed in Canada.

J   I   H   G   F   E   D   C   B

**Library of Congress Cataloging-in-Publication Data**
available from the publisher.

This book includes materials form The *Everything® Alzheimer's Book* by Carolyn Dean, M.D., © 2004, F+W Publications, Inc.

*Rite Aid Guide to Health: Alzheimer's* is intended as a reference volume only,
not as a medical manual. In light of the complex, individual, and specific
nature of heath problems, this book is not intended to replace professional
medical advice. The ideas, procedures, and suggestions in this book are
intended to supplement, not replace, the advice of a trained medical professional. Consult your physician before adopting the suggestions in this book.
The author and publisher disclaim any liability arising directly or indirectly
from the use of this book.

This publication is designed to provide accurate and authoritative information with regard to the subject matter covered. It is sold with the understanding that the publisher is not engaged in rendering legal, accounting, or other
professional advice. If legal advice or other expert assistance is required, the
services of a competent professional person should be sought.
   —From a *Declaration of Principles* jointly adopted by a Committee of the
American Bar Association and a Committee of Publishers and Associations

Many of the designations used by manufacturers and sellers to distinguish
their product are claimed as trademarks. Where those designations appear in
this book and Adams Media was aware of a trademark claim, the designations
have been printed with initial capital letters.

# Contents

# Introduction

For those of you who have been diagnosed with Alzheimer's or are caregivers of Alzheimer's patients, there are many treatments and supports that can help slow the progress of the disease and make it more bearable. Alzheimer's is not one of those diseases that you want to ignore; education about the disease is very important. The key to Alzheimer's is being aware of the warning signs and symptoms.

It is also important to obtain an early diagnosis, which can then lead to early treatment. Knowing what's available can allow you to be more interactive with your doctor and more proactive in your treatment. Early treatment can mean a much slower progression of the disease and a delay in the onset of more severe symptoms. Another ray of hope is that Alzheimer's research is moving forward at an incredible rate and the chances of a cure in the not-too-distant future are very likely. All of the information in this book will allow you to discuss options with your doctor. You'll be amazed to find out how much support there is for dealing with this very difficult condition.

*Chapter 1*

# What Is Alzheimer's?

Alzheimer's is a slow-progressing type of dementia caused by a gradual loss of brain cells. Alzheimer's disease disrupts nerve cell communication and interferes with nerve cell metabolism. As a result, damaged nerve cells can't work, can't connect, and eventually die. When nerve cells can't transmit their signals, memory fails, personality changes occur, and daily activities become impossible to perform.

## Alzheimer's—One Cause of Dementia

Dementia is a general term that describes a disease that has a set of symptoms related to a deterioration in thinking skills. Common dementia symptoms include gradual memory loss, judgment difficulties, disorientation, difficulty in learning new tasks or performing old ones, and loss of language skills. As these are also symptoms of Alzheimer's, it becomes confusing to try to differentiate between Alzheimer's and dementia, especially since people with dementia also experience personality and behavioral changes like agitation, anxiety, delusions, and hallucinations, which are also symptoms of Alzheimer's. So, in the final analysis, all people with Alzheimer's have dementia, but not all people with dementia have Alzheimer's.

In the case of Alzheimer's, the brain cells are choked off by abnormal deposits called plaques and tangles. Another characteristic of Alzheimer's is shrinkage of the brain.

The diagnosis of Alzheimer's, with an accuracy of 90 percent, is made by ruling out the different causes of dementia and by administering a highly accurate battery of neuropsychological tests. One thing we do know is that Alzheimer's is not communicable; it can't be transmitted or picked up from someone who has the disease.

Although almost 100 years have passed since identifying these plaques and tangles, an autopsy is still the only way to make a 100 percent positive diagnosis of Alzheimer's.

## The History of Alzheimer's

Alzheimer's discovery, in 1907, is credited to a German neuropathologist and clinician, Dr. Alois Alzheimer. He was the first person to describe a case of gradual mental decline of a woman he first saw in her early fifties. When she died, he equated her brain autopsy findings with her confusion and memory problems.

When first admitted to Dr. Alzheimer's psychiatric hospital in 1901, Frau Auguste D. had all the signs and symptoms of senile dementia. Because she was only fifty-one, it meant that her brain had aged ahead of her body and catapulted her thirty years into the future. Dr. Alzheimer had seen nothing like this in the past, and he watched his patient closely over the next six years as she gradually deteriorated and became bedridden.

### Frau Auguste D.'s Autopsy

When Frau Auguste D. died in 1907, Dr. Alzheimer was still at a loss to diagnosis her condition and asked to perform an autopsy on her brain. He found abnormal deposits of protein outside and inside the nerve cells in her brain, which he called neuritic plaques. Inside the cells, he found twisted and deformed fibers, which he called neurofibrillary tangles. We now know that this woman suffered from early-onset Alzheimer's, but her symptoms mimicked the gradual decline of mental function with age that was, up until that time, thought to be normal.

### Plaques and Tangles

Plaques, also called senile plaques, are the result of a buildup of a protein that is normally produced around nerve cells. In the case of Alzheimer's, however, this protein, called beta amyloid, keeps on building. Symptoms begin when the excess protein actually prevents electrical signals from being transmitted from one nerve cell to the next.

Tangles have their own story. They occur inside the nerve cell and are a buildup of another protein with the seemingly innocuous name "tau." They build up to the extent that they cause cell death and also impede the passage of information between nerve cells.

It wasn't until the early 1970s that neurologists began focusing their research on the brain. They realized that the plaques and tangles that Dr. Alzheimer had found in 1907 were also found in the normal aging brain but in much less profusion. They began to equate the amount of plaques and tangles with the appearance and severity of Alzheimer's.

### Alzheimer's Research

Alzheimer's was recognized in 1907, but Alzheimer's research remained dormant for many decades after Dr. Alzheimer's brilliant discovery. It was not even considered to be a major disease entity until the 1970s. At that time, neurological research expanded, and tremendous amounts of Dr. Alzheimer's plaques and tangles were found in patients that were thought to have dementia or senility.

**What did this discovery mean for Alzheimer's research?**

This gave hope to people who had been convinced that aging and senility went hand in hand. By distinguishing Alzheimer's as a disease separate from normal symptoms of aging, researchers could now hope to find a cure.

In the 1970s, researchers named the condition after Dr. Alzheimer since he had been the first person to equate its symptoms with plaques and tangles. Even after Alzheimer's disease was distinguished from senility and dementia by its name, it still wasn't recognized by the government for purposes of research funding. It was, however, being recognized by the families of Alzheimer's sufferers.

## The High Cost of Alzheimer's

The tremendous physical and emotional cost of the disease to Alzheimer's sufferers and their families has been known for decades. There is also, however, a financial cost of the disease. Finally, in 1998 and again in 2002, reports were commissioned by the Alzheimer's Association on the costs to U.S. businesses. Both studies were shocking.

"Alzheimer's Disease: The Costs to U.S. Businesses," authored by Ross Koppel, Ph.D., of the Social Research Corporation and the Department of Sociology at the University of Pennsylvania, found that the 2002 Alzheimer's cost to U.S. businesses would be in excess of $61 billion. To put that number into perspective, this amount is equal to the net profits of the top ten *Fortune* 500 companies and exactly double the amount that was calculated in the 1998 report. The costs to businesses to cover medical insurance and disability for workers with Alzheimer's was $24.6 billion. The costs incurred are due to the extensive responsibilities family members assume when a loved one is diagnosed with Alzheimer's. $36.5 billion of the estimated $61 billion cost is due to absenteeism, productivity losses, and labor replacement costs.

This seems like a huge amount of money until you realize that 70 percent of people with Alzheimer's live at home, where almost 75 percent of their care is organized and provided by family and friends. The remaining 25 percent, averaging $12,500 per year, is paid for by families out of their own pocket for private home care. It seems like U.S. business is subsidizing home care for Alzheimer's sufferers, but is it a less expensive option than nursing home care? The average cost for nursing home care is $42,000 per year with a high range of $70,000 per year in some areas of the country.

### It's Only Going to Get Worse

In a 1994 report from the *American Journal of Public Health* on the economical and social costs of Alzheimer's, it was the third most expensive disease in the United States after heart disease and cancer. They reported that the average lifetime cost of care for an Alzheimer's patient is $174,000 with a two to twenty year life expectancy after diagnosis. This figure does not include the loss of wages both for the Alzheimer's sufferer or the caregiver.

The costs to Medicare were calculated for the decade beginning in 2000. For Medicare beneficiaries with Alzheimer's, the 2010 costs are expected to increase 54.5 percent, from $31.9 billion in 2000 to $49.3 billion in 2010. Medicaid expenditures for residential dementia care will have an even higher increase of 80 percent, from $18.2 billion to $33 billion in the same time period.

"Alzheimer's Disease: The Costs to U.S. Businesses" was commissioned by the Alzheimer's Association in 2002 and projected the cost of Alzheimer's into the future. The account said that within a decade there could be about 14 million baby boomers with Alzheimer's.

### Early Treatment Is the Key

As the symptoms of Alzheimer's worsen, the need for more expensive care increases. A UCLA study published in the *Journal of the American Geriatrics Society* in February 2002 found that health care costs for a high-functioning patient were about $20,000 compared with a patient with severe dementia at $35,000.

> Therefore, to cut costs, many doctors and researchers warn that we need to diagnose the condition early and institute treatment protocols that can lessen the symptoms.

### Does It Always End This Way?

Sadly, Alzheimer's does eventually lead to the inability to care for oneself, and in the later stages, brain cell death, and death. We tend to see the worst case scenario when we think of Alzheimer's; there are, however, millions of people living a comfortable life with Alzheimer's, given the proper care and support.

There are other conditions that may or may not be associated with Alzheimer's that can affect people and cause a more rapid decline in health. In other words, a heart attack or stroke may be what keeps a person from the end stages of Alzheimer's.

## *Who Is Affected?*

Men and women are equally at risk for Alzheimer's. Women, because they live longer, may make up more of the Alzheimer's population, but they are no more likely to be stricken with Alzheimer's than men. Although Alzheimer's rarely occurs under age fifty, by age sixty, 2 percent of the population has Alzheimer's—that means two out of every 100 people are affected. By age eighty-five, the incidence increases to 50 percent, or five out of ten people.

## *The Risk Factors*

We know that aging is the number one risk factor for Alzheimer's. And except for the ApoE4 lipoprotein gene, Alzheimer's is not specifically a genetic disorder. The lipoprotein gene needs to be triggered or "turned on" by one or more of the following risk factors that are themselves associated with Alzheimer's.

This is the part of diagnosing Alzheimer's that is very frustrating for researchers and doctors. Alzheimer's doesn't seem to have one specific cause that you can immediately point your finger at and say "ah ha." The disease may have several contributing factors:

- Head trauma and stroke
- High-fat diet
- Chronic stress

## The Warning Signs

With the level of Alzheimer's awareness in our society, we are very attentive to when we have incidental memory lapses. With Alzheimer's, however, it's a constellation of symptoms including a confusion and disorientation that make us befuddled and apathetic, and so we may just deny it for a time. That's why it's important to be aware of the warning signs of Alzheimer's in yourself, in your parents, and in your friends.

### Mind and Memory Problems

Because nerve transmission is the first thing to deteriorate in Alzheimer's, we lose the connection to our thoughts. Everything we do in life is preceded by a thought. Most people don't vocalize their intent to do something, but if we did, it would be something like this: I think I'll get up and have a glass of water in the kitchen; while there, I see the plants need watering, too, and I'll do that; then I notice the garbage can is full, and I must change the bag.

We think of something, and it triggers us to take an action. In Alzheimer's, the thought is initiated, but it often doesn't go far enough along the nerve pathways to trigger an action before it stops dead.

The mind and memory symptoms will appear as if the memory is failing, when you can't remember a name or an event. The inability to find the right word to name a familiar object is another of Alzheimer's problems, which has to do with language. For instance, you may be able to describe what the broom does, but unable to say "broom."

Abstract thinking, which is necessary for balancing your checkbook or when you make analogies or comparisons, becomes almost impossible because of all the electrical connections that have to take place to compare one idea to another. There can even be a disconnection in recognizing your surroundings or what time of day it is. You may go to the mall and then become confused as to where you are. Because you forget what you are doing, you can leave the stove turned on or the kettle boiling dry, and this is often interpreted as poor judgment.

### Difficulty Doing Things

The electrical disconnection of Alzheimer's makes it very difficult to accomplish tasks, even if you have done them for a lifetime. You think a thought and really want to do something, like make a cup of tea or pick up the mail, but the electrical connections between thinking the thought and performing the action just won't work. With Alzheimer's, you think of something and you may even begin a task, but then not remember what you are doing midtask and stop in your tracks. As the disease progresses, you may not even have enough memory connections to begin the task. Too many cells are tangled up and blocked by plaque to make the connection. You may pick up the mail because it came through the mail slot and is lying on the floor, but when you look at it you may not know what it is or what to do with it. Or, you may start putting the tea bags in the freezer or your keys in the cat box.

### Mood and Behavior Problems

Memory lapses and the misplacement of things are often easy to deny, but when irritability, agitation, and depression begin to descend, you know something is wrong. By the very nature of mood changes and rapid mood swings, however, you often drive away family and friends from getting close enough to find out what's really going on. And it's not just the irritability and depression that are signs of Alzheimer's; it's also the fear. It's a very scary thing to feel you are "losing your mind." That's the very time you really need all the love and support you can gather around you. So, be aware that you might be driving away your support team.

Your family may say you seem different. They may pick up the personality changes that set in because of the memory loss and inability to complete tasks. Understandably, you may be confused and suspicious. You become fearful and either push people away and refuse their help or become dependent and won't let them out of your sight.

Over 4.5 million Americans have Alzheimer's—that's 25 percent of all the cases in the world. But the United States only makes up 4.6 percent of the world's population.

The electrical disconnection in the brain also causes apathy to set in. The last thing you want to do is to start a conversation, go out, or get involved in a social activity.

# Chapter 2

# Alzheimer's: The Differential Diagnosis

Nobody wants to wait for an autopsy to obtain a diagnosis, but that's the state of the art in Alzheimer's. When you first start to have memory loss, you, like Ronald Reagan, may laugh it off for a few years. And with luck, you may just be experiencing normal signs of aging where a few brain cells go down for the count. Family doctors, however, should be alerted to signs of Alzheimer's so that treatment can be started as early as possible.

## Early Detection of Symptoms

You know something is wrong because you've put your house keys in the freezer once too often. At first it was a joke, even though you didn't share it with anyone because you knew they would think it was a bit crazy. But then you got confused at the shopping mall parking lot the other day and couldn't find your car for the longest time. That was scary. And, even though you told her there is nothing wrong, your daughter keeps saying that you are more irritable and even paranoid lately. What's going on?

It is a scary feeling when your mind goes blank and you can't remember where you are or what you are doing. Because these feelings come and go in Alzheimer's, you don't really pay attention to them. This slow deterioration of brain cells causes intermittent interruption of signals. The next day can be perfectly normal because the signals all go through, and you can tell yourself that everything is fine. Such is the power of denial.

Chances are that your family doctor will be the first doctor to consider the diagnosis of Alzheimer's. But, he or she may not be the first person to recognize the signs and symptoms.

That person is usually a spouse or another family member.

Someone who hasn't seen you for a few months or a year will usually be the first to notice a change in your personality or your level of functioning. Family that sees you every day or every week may not even notice a slow progression of symptoms. And everyone, doctors included, is very quick to dismiss memory problems, saying, "Oh, you're getting on in years, you know." Only someone who saw you do crossword puzzles last year and now sees that you can't remember where you put your glasses begins to raise the alarm.

Fear of finding out that you have Alzheimer's is the main reason why you may delay your first visit to your doctor. But you must remember that knowledge is power. In the case of Alzheimer's, the sooner you know, the sooner you can do something about it.

You will probably see your family doctor and blurt out the question, "Do I have Alzheimer's?" Your doctor may be taken off guard, but if he or she has seen some deterioration in your mental status over the past years, then you have opened the door to finding out why you feel the way you do.

## It's a Matter of Exclusion

Even before you finish your sentence, your doctor is running through a list of what other conditions could cause your symptoms. In order to diagnose Alzheimer's, your doctor has to exclude all those other conditions based on your history, physical and neurological tests, lab tests, and scans. Because to definitively diagnose Alzheimer's you have to wait for an autopsy, your doctor must rule out all other possibilities before he or she says you have Alzheimer's. The process of doing this is called differential diagnosis. Alzheimer's disease is a type of dementia that may be difficult to distinguish from many other conditions. Some of these other causes of dementia may be more treatable than Alzheimer's:

- Senility and dementia
- Organic brain syndrome
- Cardiovascular disorders
- Trauma-induced brain injury
- Metabolic disorders
- Prescription drugs and drug interactions

## Senility and Dementia

Senility and dementia are still considered by many to be a normal stage of aging. They are catchall diagnoses and are freely used to diagnose any memory symptoms in the elderly. With age, we assume that most people will lose some important brain cells and decline in mental function.

The definition of senile is as follows: forgetful, confused, or otherwise mentally less acute in later life; occurring in or believed to be characteristic of later life, especially the period after the age of sixty-five years.

The definition of senile dementia is: A form of brain disorder marked by progressive and irreversible mental deterioration, memory loss, and disorientation, known to affect some people after the age of about sixty-five years.

What an irony that the age of retirement is also designated as the age when senility sets in.

## Organic Brain Syndrome

Organic brain syndrome (OBS) is a general term used to designate diseases that affect mental status. The organic part refers to a physical disease or condition that affects the brain and causes a decrease in mental function. Psychiatric disorders are not included in the organic brain syndrome category. Symptoms vary for different diseases, but in general include confusion, delirium, dementia, and agitation.

OBS is a disease of the elderly. It's as if the brain just gets rusty with age and slows down. But OBS is not inevitable as you grow older. There are many disorders associated with OBS. Many of them can present symptoms similar to Alzheimer's because Alzheimer's disease is also a degenerative neurological disorder; these disorders must be ruled out in the differential diagnosis.

### Creutzfeldt-Jakob: Mad Cow Disease

This disease is a rapidly progressing OBS that affects mental function and movement. It is characterized by brain destruction due to a viral-like protein particle called a prion, which can be transmitted from an infected living creature to humans. It's very rare, and occurs in only two per one million people. The average age of onset of this disease is fifty.

Creutzfeldt-Jakob distinguishes itself from Alzheimer's because of the rapidly fatal progression of the disease. It begins with personality changes and poor coordination and progresses to severe dementia, muscle tremors, and rigid posture.

Live transplants, such as corneal transplants, from patients who have the disease carry a potential for the disease. A family history of dementia is also a risk factor.

More has become known about Creutzfeldt-Jakob disease because of the British, and now the American, experience with mad cow disease. Creutzfeldt-Jakob disease may be related to other prion diseases including kuru (documented in New Guinea headhunters), scrapie (found in sheep), and bovine spongiform encephalitis (seen in cows).

### Huntington's Chorea

This OBS is also rare, and affects five in one million. It's an inherited condition caused by a gene mutation. Huntington's Chorea causes degeneration of the nerve cells in the cerebrum. It resembles Alzheimer's in the personality changes, progressive loss of mental function, and loss of cognitive functions such as speech, calculative skills, and judgment.

It was first described by an American doctor, George Huntington, in 1872. It wasn't until 1993, however, that a team of researchers at the Massachusetts Institute of Technology (MIT) found the gene responsible for this disease on chromosome number four. It is unlike Alzheimer's because symptoms appear from age thirty-five to fifty even though the gene is present from birth.

Huntingon's Chorea causes dementia, but unlike Alzheimer's, it is a hereditary condition. If one parent has the gene, then half of his or her children will have the condition. It also differs from Alzheimer's because it is characterized by frequent abnormal facial and body movements, which include quick jerking movements. Chorea means "dance" and refers to the puppet-like jerking of the body.

### Multiple Sclerosis

Multiple sclerosis (MS) is an OBS that involves the brain and the spinal cord. It's a disease that causes scarring or sclerosis of the myelin sheath that covers all the nerve cells in the body. Six out of ten cases affect women, and it is fairly common, occurring in one out of 1,600 people. It is not an "elderly disease" and arises between the ages of twenty and forty. In people under sixty-five, MS is a major cause of disability.

It comes about with repeated episodes of inflammation of nervous tissue in any area of the brain and spinal cord. The inflammation can affect vision, movement, or sensation, and is different in each person. The scarring of various nerves slows or blocks the transmission of nerve impulses in the inflamed area, which results in typical MS symptoms.

We know MS is caused by inflammation, but we don't know what triggers the inflammation in the first place. Researchers theorize that it is triggered by a type of viral infection or some gene abnormality that controls the immune system, or a combination of both.

### Normal Pressure Hydrocephalus (NPH)

This OBS occurs when the normal flow of cerebral spinal fluid (CSF) is blocked. With no way to get out, it builds up and enlarges the ventricles within the brain, and the pressure it puts on adjacent brain tissue causes tissue destruction. As we are finding out, any damage to delicate brain tissue can lead to symptoms of dementia. This condition occurs in one out of 100,000 people and can be reversed or treated if properly diagnosed.

Some risk factors and causes of NPH are head injury, brain surgery, meningitis, and brain hemorrhage. The pressure often diminishes when the swelling subsides over time with these conditions. In addition, a temporary "shunt," or drainage tube, can be put in the brain to release the excess CSF build up.

## *Pick's Disease*

Pick's disease is also called presenile dementia because it occurs in younger adults. In this condition, brain atrophy occurs and on autopsy, abnormal bodies (Pick's bodies) are present in the nerve cells usually in the frontal or temporal lobes of the brain. It is another rare disorder affecting one out of 100,000 people.

Pick's disease is more common in women and may be evident in people as young as twenty but usually begins between forty and sixty years of age. It differs from Alzheimer's because there are no plaques or tangles to be seen, but patients have Alzheimer's-like symptoms. The cause of Pick's disease is unknown but thought to be a genetic disorder.

## *Parkinson's Disease*

This is a much more common disorder than many of the other neurological diseases we have been talking about. It occurs in two out of 1,000 people, but unlike Alzheimer's, it develops early, around the age of fifty. Both men and women are affected equally, and it is becoming one of the most common diseases of the nervous system in the over-fifty population.

With this disease, movement is impaired, which makes walking difficult. There is also a general shaking of the head and hands and loss of coordination. Like Alzheimer's, there is progressive damage of nerve cells, but in Parkinson's the damage is confined to nerve cells in an area of the brain that controls movement. Dopamine, a neurotransmitter from these cells, is consequently diminished and produces loss of muscle function. As with Alzheimer's, we really don't know why the cells are destroyed in the first place. Dementia is a symptom of later-stage Parkinson's. Some of the drug treatments for Parkinson's, however, may cause dementia.

### Lung Disorders and Alcohol-Related Conditions

There are several lung disorders that may cause or aggravate OBS simply because not enough oxygen is getting to the brain. Sleep apnea is an increasingly common condition in which breathing stops for several seconds and oxygen to the brain is reduced. Emphysema may also lower the oxygen supply to the brain. All of these conditions can cause symptoms of confusion and even memory loss that could be misinterpreted as dementia by the casual observer.

Alcohol-induced dementia is called Wernicke-Korsakoff syndrome. The underlying cause is a vitamin B1 deficiency caused by malnutrition common in habitual alcohol use. Wernicke-Korsakoff syndrome affects people between forty and eighty years old with a gradual onset. Symptoms are often reversible, however, especially in the early stages, with high doses of vitamin B1.

## Cardiovascular Disorders

The heart and blood vessels are responsible for transporting oxygen-rich and glucose-rich blood to all parts of the body. So, it's obvious that when the heart and blood vessels are impaired or damaged, they can't get enough oxygen or glucose to the brain. Lack of oxygen to the brain for over four minutes can result in death. Shorter periods of no oxygen or prolonged low levels of oxygen can result in nerve cell death in the brain, and in symptoms such as dementia.

The following cardiovascular disorders can result in impaired blood flow to the brain.

**Arrhythmias:** A disturbance of the electrical conduction system of the heart that interrupts the heart rate or rhythm. When the heart beats too fast or too slow and the flow of blood to the brain is impaired for even a few seconds, brain damage can occur.

**Cardiac Infections:** A bacterial or viral infection of the inside lining of the heart, which can impair blood flow to the brain.

**Multi-Infarct Dementia (MID):** MID affects four out of 10,000 people and accounts for 10–20 percent of all dementias. It happens when atherosclerotic cholesterol plaque in arteries breaks off and blocks off small blood vessels in the brain causing tissue death.

**Stroke:** Stroke is usually caused by a blood clot or buildup of cholesterol plaque that blocks an artery in the brain. Depending on where it occurs, it can mimic any and all symptoms of dementia. The incidence of stroke is about four out of 1,000 people; it is the third leading cause of death in the United States. Risk for stroke includes high blood pressure, heart disease, smoking, high cholesterol, and diabetes.

**Transient Ischemic Attack (TIA):** TIAs are also called mini-strokes, and are defined as blood flow disruption and decreased brain function for less than twenty-four hours at a time.

## Trauma-Induced Brain Injury

Motor vehicle accidents, sports trauma, bike accidents, and serious falls can all result in head injuries that cause swelling and bleeding; this puts pressure on delicate brain tissue, and sometimes results in symptoms of dementia. Of course, you should remember if you have had a head injury, and suspect any mental impairment could be due to that. Sometimes, however, the symptoms come long after a traumatic event.

Even a minor trauma, when combined with taking blood thinners or aspirin or alcohol intake will thin the blood and could turn a minor bleed into a major one. The symptoms may come on so gradually that the trauma and the symptoms are not connected.

The result of delayed treatment could be dementia-like symptoms due to chronic subdural hematoma, intracerebral hemorrhage, subarachnoid hemorrhage, or a concussion.

## Metabolic Disorders

Disorders of metabolism can produce chemicals in the body that are toxic to the brain. This form of dementia occurs in about one in 10,000 people. This type of dementia may be reversible and deserves a close investigation by your doctor. Outright liver and kidney failure can cause dementia but are usually not reversible.

## *Endocrine Disorders*

Metabolic causes of dementia may include endocrine disorders such as:

- **Addison's disease:** failure of the adrenal glands.
- **Cushing's disease:** overproduction of adrenal hormone.
- **Diabetic nephropathy:** diabetic kidney disease.
- **Diabetic ketoacidosis:** overproduction of ketones.
- **Insulinoma causing hypoglycemia:** low blood sugar.
- **Hypoglycemia:** low blood sugar.
- **Hypoparathyroidism:** imbalance of calcium in the body.
- **Hyperparathyroidism:** imbalance of calcium in the body.
- **Hypothyroidism:** low thyroid hormone.
- **Thyrotoxicosis:** overproduction of thyroid hormone.
- **Pheochromocytoma:** overproduction of adrenalin.

## *Electrolyte Imbalance and Nutritional Deficiency*

Metabolic disorders causing dementia can manifest as disorders of electrolytes creating acid/base disorders, low sodium, high calcium, low potassium, and low magnesium. Nutritional disorders such as vitamin B1 deficiency, vitamin B12 deficiency, niacin deficiency, and protein-calorie malnutrition can produce dementia. Studies show that the majority of nursing home patients are malnourished and deficient in most vitamins.

# Prescription Drugs and Drug Interactions

Prescription medication may cause toxic OBS. There is, of course, a scientific basis with each prescription drug tested in extensive clinical trials. Most drug research subjects, however, are healthy, white males. A drug may pass all the tests required for it to become an FDA-approved medication, but it's not until the drug gets into the general population that it is used by all ages.

In the elderly, however, drug metabolism is usually slower, which means it takes longer for a certain amount of medication to clear the body. The bowels move slower; the digestion is slower; the liver doesn't work at top speed. Therefore, if high drug doses are given to an elderly person, there is the potential of a toxic drug reaction. Seniors often also take multiple prescriptions; this creates a complexity of drug interactions that may cause toxic OBS. Nearly one quarter of our elderly are admitted to hospitals or nursing homes because of medication side effects.

*Chapter 3*

# Your Physical Examination

Annual physical exams include the standard: taking your blood pressure, listening to your heart and lungs, tapping your knees, and then you are out the door. Maybe every few years you get some blood tests for hemoglobin or cholesterol, but they are often within normal range. A physical exam is pretty basic, unless your doctor is looking for something specific. That's why you almost have to prod your doctor into checking you for Alzheimer's.

## Medical History and Physical Exam

Because a definite diagnosis of Alzheimer's can only be done after an autopsy, the only way to diagnosis a living person with Alzheimer's is by excluding a list of other possibilities, through a process called differential diagnosis. Some of these other causes of dementia are often mistaken for and may be more treatable than Alzheimer's:

- Senility and dementia
- Organic brain syndrome
- Cardiovascular disorders
- Trauma-induced brain injury
- Metabolic disorders
- Prescription drugs and drug interactions

If you ask your doctor about Alzheimer's, your doctor will take a medical history and find out when you first started having memory problems, confusion, and personality changes, all done so with a list of forms of dementia in the forefront of his or her mind. You will be asked about any past head trauma, surgery, medication, and exposure to toxic chemicals. Then your doctor will ask for a detailed family history, which includes any family member who has or had neurological disease.

If he or she does suspect some neurological disease, you will also be referred to a specialist. In the meantime, your doctor will do the following examination.

**General appearance:** Look for apathetic appearance and flat stare to rule out Parkinson's disease.

**General appearance:** Nutritional status—check for dehydration, muscle wasting, bruising, brittle hair and nails, and dry skin.

**Eyes:** Perform an eye examination to rule out brain tumors, which cause pressure that can be seen at the back of your eye.

**Head:** Test your cranial nerves to rule out brain tumors.

**Neck:** Feel your thyroid to help diagnose hypothyroidism or hyperthyroidism.

**Heart:** Check your heart sounds, pulse, and blood pressure to help rule out arrhythmias, valve problems, and hypertension.

**Lungs:** Listen to your lungs to help rule out lung disease.

**Reflexes:** Test your reflexes to help rule out other neurological diseases.

**Abdomen:** Feel your liver to rule out liver disease.

## The Neurologist

If your family doctor suspects you may have a neurological disease, he or she will probably send you to see a neurologist to help decide on your diagnosis. Neurologists have standard tests for memory, reasoning, vision-motor coordination, and language skills. Researchers are working hard to improve a series of standardized tests that can be given to people at risk in order to detect early Alzheimer's or to predict whether you are at a higher risk of developing Alzheimer's in the future. These tests are also used to monitor the progression of Alzheimer's.

The first examination the neurologist administers will become the baseline test. The current tests in use include the Mini-Mental State Examination (MMSE) or Physical Self-Maintenance Scale (PSMS).

They assess cognition (thinking) and function. To begin, you may be asked what day, month, and year it is, followed by more and more difficult questions. You'll be asked to name common items from pictures and maybe to use building blocks to reconstruct drawings of block structures. It does sound a bit like preschool, but these simple tests give important information about how the brain is functioning.

Other neurological tests for sensation, balance, and temperature are carried out. Then decisions have to be made about scans and laboratory tests. Usually a brain scan is done to detect other causes of dementia such as stroke. Laboratory tests can help exclude metabolic diseases, organ diseases, and endocrine diseases.

### Alzheimer's Testing

Alzheimer's testing is focused in several areas. There is no one definitive test for the condition, so it becomes a process of excluding other possible conditions, doing intensive memory and language tests, and performing more and more sophisticated brain scanning technology. Testing for Alzheimer's includes memory and language tests, tests for existing brain damage and its association with Alzheimer's, tests for blood chemistry changes and the association with Alzheimer's, and neuroimaging.

## I'd Still Rather Not Know

Every day research comes to light with new information about Alzheimer's disease. There are, however, other practical benefits to an early diagnosis. Sometimes it's just good to know that there is something physical going on, and even a bad diagnosis is still a diagnosis.

The sooner you and your family know that you have Alzheimer's, the more time you have to plan for the future. It's just wise to make financial decisions, think about living arrangements and power of attorney, and create your support system early on.

### *Possible or Probable Alzheimer's*

When you get your final diagnosis from your doctor it will be couched in one of two terms, Possible, or Probable, Alzheimer's. Probable Alzheimer's means your doctor has tried to rule out all other dementia disorders and has concluded that your symptoms are probably due to Alzheimer's. The less precise diagnosis of Possible Alzheimer's implies that even though Alzheimer's is likely the main cause of your dementia, there may be one or more other conditions that are causing similar symptoms and possibly making your Alzheimer's symptoms appear worse.

### *Documenting the Progression of Alzheimer's*

Though we don't know what causes Alzheimer's, we have been able to discover what happens in the brain when Alzheimer's attacks, and to correlate it with progressive physical and mental changes.

There has been a concerted effort to document the progression of symptoms in Alzheimer's disease in stages in order to determine medical treatment options, and to assess home care and long-term care needs.

**How long after a diagnosis of Alzheimer's does a patient have left to live?**

In a late diagnosis, the time until death can be as short as three years, especially in patients over age eighty, or as long as ten years or more in younger patients.

Progression of Alzheimer's symptoms seems to follow the buildup of plaques and tangles and nerve cell degeneration in the brain. We know that plaque first builds up near, and then in, the hippocampus, the memory center. Plaque may, however, appear a full ten to twenty years before any actual symptoms begin. As plaque builds and spreads, memory is affected first, and then slowly but inexorably, all aspects of behavior, thinking, and judgment are affected. The final stages involve the areas of movement and coordination, causing immobility.

## The Seven Stages of Alzheimer's

Doctors commonly assign Alzheimer's symptoms to one of the following three stages: mild, moderate, or severe. These will be compared with the more precise Seven Stages of Alzheimer's.

**Stage 1:** No cognitive impairment.

**Stage 2:** Very mild cognitive decline; forgetfulness.

**Stage 3:** Mild cognitive decline; early confusional state.

**Stage 4:** Moderate cognitive decline (mild stage); late confusional state.

**Stage 5:** Moderately severe cognitive decline (moderate stage); early dementia.

**Stage 6:** Severe cognitive decline (moderately severe stage); middle dementia.

**Stage 7:** Very severe cognitive decline (severe stage); late dementia.

No two people experience the same degree of symptoms or even fall clearly into one stage or another at any one time. The purpose of staging in Alzheimer's is not to force people into one category or another; it's to help give the patient, the doctor, and the caregivers a clear picture of how the disease is progressing.

### Stage 1: No Cognitive Impairment

This designation implies that we are all at Stage 1 Alzheimer's, with no noticeable symptoms. Sixty percent of the general population has the ApoE4 gene that creates a susceptibility to Alzheimer's. Many of us are at risk for stroke or have high levels of homocysteine, which also increases our risk for Alzheimer's. This is the stage where lifestyle intervention, in the form of a good diet, exercise, and certain nutrients, could mean the difference between health and Alzheimer's. This is the stage in the brain where plaques and tangles could start to build up, but take ten to twenty years to be recognized as impaired memory.

### Stage 2: Very Mild Cognitive Decline

This is the memory lapse stage. Names, keys, and glasses disappear in the twinkling of an eye. It's a stage that is equated with aging, being stressed, or having too much on your plate, and for many people this is exactly what is happening.

Even if you mention memory lapse to your doctor, he or she usually doesn't think it's important, and no one else seems to notice. It's not even denial at this stage; it's just part of life. If you do go on to develop full-blown Alzheimer's, this stage is equated with the increasing buildup of plaques and tangles in the brain.

### Stage 3: Mild Cognitive Decline

This stage corresponds with Mild Alzheimer's. Your family and friends remark on your memory problems. Physically, you are just fine. What's happening in your brain is beginning to affect memory, language, and reasoning, but has not reached your movement centers.

A diagnosis of Possible Alzheimer's, however, could be made at this time based on detailed mental status testing. The symptoms are all mild, but if you put them all together, they form an undeniable pattern. Symptoms that stand out include: problems remembering names or finding the right word, inability to remember reading material, losing important things, inability to plan or organize, taking a long time with tasks, inability to perform effectively at work, and a growing sense of anxiety.

> This disease gives no early physical clues. Yet, you are finding it more and more difficult to keep your world in control. You may just liken your symptoms to normal aging at this time.

### Stage 4: Moderate Cognitive Decline

Mild Alzheimer's encompasses Stages 3 and 4. In Stage 4, even a cursory medical examination would detect neurological deficits. Personality changes become obvious at this stage, with the most common being shy and withdrawn behavior, especially in groups of people.

Symptoms that stand out at this stage are a decreased knowledge or awareness of current events, difficulty counting backward from 100 by sevens, difficulty making a shopping list and shopping, making mistakes in paying bills and managing finances, forgetting aspects of personal history, getting lost in familiar places, making bad decisions through bad judgment, loss of spontaneity, and mood changes.

### Stage 5: Moderately Severe Cognitive Decline

This is the Moderate Alzheimer's stage. This stage shows evidence of major memory gaps and obvious problems with thinking, language, and tasks. In the brain, plaques and tangles have spread from the hippocampus memory center and are increasing in the areas of the cerebral cortex that control thought, language, reasoning, and sensory processing. As the cells are damaged and killed, they create areas of atrophy that can be diagnosed with a brain scan.

In Stage 5 Alzheimer's, the problems are such that some daily caregiving and support are essential. The Alzheimer's patient may forget addresses and telephone numbers but will know children's or spouse's names. There will be additional symptoms such as confusion as to time and place; confusion that is worse at sundown; agitation, restlessness, anxiety, and crying; inability to cope with new situations or stress; inability to count backward by twos from forty; problems with reading and writing; a very short attention span; inability to think logically; inability to dress appropriately for weather or events; and inability to eat or use the bathroom unassisted.

### Stage 6: Severe Cognitive Decline

On the Mild, Moderate, to Severe Alzheimer's scale, Stage 6 is Moderately Severe. At this stage, symptoms are obviously worsening in memory and personality. The amount of care needed is increased to cover all activities of daily living. Behavior problems, such as wandering and agitation, are common. More intensive supervision and care are necessary to prevent wandering or dangerous activities such as leaving the stove turned on or leaving doors and windows open.

This is the stage when local services should be called in to help the family. Alzheimer's sufferers in Stage 6 may be unaware of their surroundings or recent experiences; have great difficulty remembering personal history; may still remember their own name; may forget a spouse's name but seem to know familiar faces; must be assisted getting dressed; experience sleep disturbances; must be assisted in the bathroom; begin experiencing urinary or fecal incontinence; express major personality changes and behavioral symptoms such as suspiciousness, delusions, hallucinations, and compulsive, repetitive behaviors; forget where they are and wander away and get lost; have little to no impulse control and may undress at inappropriate times or places or use vulgar language; or have trouble getting out of a chair.

### Stage 7: Very Severe Cognitive Decline

This is the Severe stage of Alzheimer's; this final stage includes loss of all contact with the outside world, inability to respond or speak coherently, and inability to move. In the brain, plaques and tangles are widespread, leaving devastation and atrophy. Symptoms are those of total incapacity, and patients need assistance in eating and going to the bathroom; in addition, they have incontinence; are unable to walk, sit, smile, or hold their head up; their only vocalizations are groaning, moaning, or grunting; muscles become rigid; swallowing is impaired; they experience weight loss and seizures; have skin infections; and sleep for long periods.

## How Alzheimer's Patients Succumb

Due to lack of activity and prolonged confinement to bed, most Alzheimer's patients die from other diseases. One frequent cause of death is pneumonia, either after a cold or flu, or due to aspiration of food into the lungs because of impaired swallowing.

No, it's not a pretty sight; it's not anything our loved ones or we should go through. That is why it's important to have all the facts about Alzheimer's, find all the sufferers, and do all the research necessary to find a cure to stop this tragedy.

# Chapter 4

# Coping with the Diagnosis

Coping with a diagnosis of Alzheimer's is a matter of making the best of a bad situation and marking time until a treatment plan is proven to halt the disease. It's not as if you'll be lying back and waiting for the end to come. Coping isn't a passive activity when it comes to Alzheimer's. There are a million things for you to do to plan for your best possible future.

## Bringing Out the Best

It's been said many times that we rise to our highest potential when faced with adversity. When faced with the diagnosis of Alzheimer's, we are certainly put to the test. You begin by finding out all you can about the disease and doing what you can to maintain your health. Then you must come to grips with the fact that within a decade, your mind is not going to be able to make decisions. You have to make ten times the decisions now to make up for not being able to do so in the future.

> You have to plan your future so you can spend your years with an appreciation of life and gather a support team around that will give you comfort, dignity, and respect.

## Bringing Out the Worst

There is also no set way of coping with Alzheimer's. You might feel like this diagnosis is the straw that breaks the camel's back, and you just can't cope with it. It may feel like you are being punished and bring up the "why me" question. The following stages of grieving may begin to play out in your head. They are presented in a linear order, but you can go in and out of several of the stages at one time before you reach acceptance. Dr. Elisabeth Kübler-Ross, in her work *On Death and Dying*, was the first to define the stages of grieving as:

- Denial
- Anger
- Bargaining
- Depression
- Acceptance

### *Denial*

You've probably become quite good at denial for the past few years about the true nature of your symptoms. There is something to be said for denying minor aches and pains and getting on with life. But, if you have really made all efforts to make sure the diagnosis is accurate, now is the time to accept it. Now is the time to put your energy and attention on living the best life you can.

### Anger

Anger is a normal reaction. It is good to express your true feelings at this stage and not bottle them up. By holding back strong emotions, you can actually cause more stress and physical symptoms. But, there's a time to put anger aside. Work with a counselor to express your feelings of anger and come to terms with them.

### Bargaining

Bargaining is an internal process that usually occurs when you are alone and praying for a miracle. For some, bargaining with God takes the form of promising you'll be a better person, devote yourself to service, become a priest, a nun, or a Mother Teresa if only this punishment will be lifted.

### Depression

A level of depression is probably with you when you first suspect you have Alzheimer's. And you have a right to be depressed. If you have a history of depression, this type of bad news will further burden you. With support and counseling, however, you can strive to keep yourself from feeling weighed down and find some joy in life.

### Acceptance

Acceptance is the final stage in the process of grieving, and most people do get to it. Sometimes it comes in a flash of understanding, after a period of prayer and meditation. You learn that the reason, or the lesson, or the need for you to have this terrible condition does not matter, and you say, "So be it!"

Some people even get to see the gift in the tragedy. Families can become reunited, and resources that you never realized were in yourself or others, surface. Acceptance is the state that will help you stay the healthiest and make your caregiver's work that much easier.

### Creating a Checklist

A part of acceptance is planning a course of action now that you know you have Alzheimer's.

The checklist that you must make is one that can branch out into many different areas. It covers your whole life. Following it through can make your future as comfortable as possible.

- ✓ Talk with your family about your future needs regarding long-term home care and future nursing care.

- ✓ If you work, talk with your employer or employees.

- ✓ Join a local Alzheimer's support group.

- ✓ Discuss your health insurance with your insurance agent.

- ✓ Discuss your finances with a financial advisor or banking counselor.

- ✓ Talk to a lawyer about who you want to have your power of attorney and to be executor of your estate.

- ✓ Alzheimer's-proof your house.

- ✓ Talk to an Alzheimer's counselor about when you should stop driving.

## Take Care of Your Health

During the times when you are depressed, you are probably not in the best frame of mind to take care of yourself. The negative self-talk floods your mind with, "Why should I take care of myself? I have Alzheimer's!"

We do know, however, that taking care of your health is the best thing to do for Alzheimer's. Consider your new job to be staying as healthy as possible until the best treatment for Alzheimer's is found.

### *Get Physical*

Take care of your physical health. See your doctor regularly to keep up on the latest Alzheimer's treatments. The best advice is to eat a healthy, low-fat, low-calorie diet and exercise daily. Take supplements and medications as directed. Keep alcohol intake to a minimum, and get eight hours of sleep a night.

### *Strengthen Your Mental Health*

Take care of your mental health. Exercise your brain as much as you do your body. Turn off the television. Join a book club; add new words to your vocabulary; and work on crossword puzzles. Start writing a diary; use big words; express yourself. A diary is also a way to write down what you need and keep lists of what you have to do as a memory jogger. Take your diary to family meetings and read from it when you forget something.

#### What about attitude?

Do your best to keep a positive mental attitude. You have a right to be down but try to realize that negative thoughts attract more negative thoughts. Being positive, especially around friends and family, will make it easier for them to do the same.

### *Support Your Emotional Health*

Take care of your emotional health. Denial, anger, fear, isolation, depression, loss of confidence, and frustration are normal emotions in your situation. Find a counselor, social worker, or psychotherapist to discuss your emotions with and to put them into perspective.

Additionally, prayer and meditation can help your emotional and spiritual health in these difficult times. Talk to a minister, priest, rabbi, or other religious advisor.

### *Just Ask*

The resources you need to take care of yourself include your family, doctors, social workers, counselors, and a support group. Creating contacts with all these support systems is important when you are first diagnosed. Don't wait until you can't fully communicate what you want from these people before asking for their assistance.

One of the hardest things for Alzheimer's patients to do is to ask for help. But we all know that life is a "give and take." You have to look at this time of your life as a time when you need to take and others have to give. You will also find that caregivers don't look upon their role as a "have to" at all. Giving from the heart is a reward in itself because it opens up the heart to receive in so many other ways.

## Talk with Your Family

Your family doesn't know what you are going through. Nobody can know exactly what you are experiencing. That's where your strength and courage come in. You can actually find yourself in the role of comforting them! When you can create a little laughter in the midst of this devastating news, your family will think you're a saint. The best is when you can mix tears of sadness and tears of laughter together; it's a wonderful combination that makes it easier for everyone to cope.

In the midst of the laughing, crying, and sharing, make sure that your family understands that it's not just an aging process that you are going through.

Additionally, your family needs to know that you require honest interaction, not a sugarcoated version of reality.

Your family needs to know that Alzheimer's is a brain disease that will impair your memory, thinking, and behavior. And there will be a time when you aren't able to take care of yourself.

You've probably been through many of life's challenges with your family and friends. Let them know that this disease will change your life and their lives, but together you can meet the challenge.

### Talk about Your Present Needs

This is a conversation apart from talking about your diagnosis and your feelings. You need to be very clear with your family about what you can and can't do. You can tell them about your plans for improving your physical, mental, emotional, and spiritual health and ask for their support. Then you need to discuss who is able to help you with:

- Meetings with your employer, insurance agent, financial advisor, and lawyer
- Doctor's appointments

- Alzheimer's-proofing your home
- Finding an Alzheimer's support group

### *Talk about Your Future Needs*

The most important thing to get clear about your future is where you will be spending it. About 70 percent of Alzheimer's sufferers are taken care of at home. With the increased government and public awareness of Alzheimer's, it is becoming easier to get assistance from the community and Alzheimer's groups. Alzheimer's support groups, caregiver training, access to the latest research, and a determination to find the "cure" are driving the Alzheimer's movement.

Discussing a time when you will be completely dependent on others is very difficult. The tables are turning. We are taken care of as infants; then we take care of our children or nieces and nephews; then we are taken care of as we decline. It happens as regularly as day flows into night. But, like death, we don't expect it to happen to us. It takes some getting used to.

### *Talk with Your Spouse*

This is a special and ongoing conversation. You and your spouse may already know about the worst aspects of Alzheimer's through the media, and you know it's going to be rough. But it's not like that in the early stages, and it's not rough all the time. You need to talk to one another about your concerns. A support group for your spouse may be very helpful.

Talking with a counselor can help answer questions about the stages of Alzheimer's and what resources you need to cope with the emotional side of losing someone who is still there beside you. Your counselor may also initiate a frank discussion about changes in intimacy and sexual relations and how you each can meet your needs.

But it's important not to live in the future. Live in the present: Take a trip; go on outings; enjoy life to the fullest. If you have no physical handicaps, there is nothing preventing you from doing all those things you always wanted to do.

Along with the rest of the family, decide on care-giving duties. You and your spouse need to make sure there is enough support, and if not, plans should be made for hiring help with housekeeping, additional caregivers, or working with Medicare for coverage.

### Talking with Children and Teens

Children and teens, whether you are their parent or grandparent, are going to have a whole different take on what's happening than adults. They can't be expected to know what the disease is all about, and may think you're going "crazy."

For teens, showing them a picture of the cross section of a brain and telling them that a disease is damaging your brain may help them understand. Younger children mainly want reassurances. They can feel something is shifting in the family dynamic. Hugging and holding them is the best thing. Reassure young children that they cannot "catch" the disease from you.

Explain to preadolescent kids that you have a disease where you are going to forget things, even their names, and that you still love them very much. You must decide whether the school nurse and teachers should know about your illness. There are also Alzheimer's support groups especially for children and teens. Stay involved in important future events in your children's or grandchildren's lives. Write letters or make audio or videotapes with your advice, thoughts, and feelings about their first date, their graduation, their marriage, and even your death.

## Talk with Others

Once you have discussed Alzheimer's with your family, you will need to inform others. While this may make you feel uncomfortable or embarrassed, preparations need to be made and people need to be informed.

### Talk with Your Boss, Coworkers, or Employees

Many Alzheimer's workers are reducing their workload, taking early retirement, and eventually going on long-term disability. But because

Alzheimer's is becoming more common, many employers are working on their own coping strategies. Speaking directly about your limitations is important in order to create the best possible working relationship.

You may need less of a workload and someone to assist you so that you can do what you do best, and not have to rely on short-term memory if that is your biggest challenge. It's going to be difficult to speak about your limitations, but it's better than doing a bad job and trying to cover it up.

### Discuss Insurance, Finances, and Legal Matters

These three aspects of your future are crucial to take care of as soon as possible. You need to know how much your current health insurance will cover, and whether you need to apply for Medicare or Medicaid. Your finances have to be organized so that someone else can take them over for you when it becomes necessary. If you own a home, you have to decide whether or not to transfer it over to a family member. And you have to decide on power of attorney and the executor of your estate. These are all thorny matters in the best of times. Sitting with professionals who do this every day is the key to doing it right.

### *Join a Local Alzheimer's Support Group*

Most communities have Alzheimer's support groups either connected to a local hospital or run by a volunteer agency such as the Alzheimer's Association. These are groups that will welcome you with open arms from a place of great caring and sharing. They are there so you don't have to reinvent the wheel when it comes to what needs to be done for your care and support for your family.

*Chapter 5*

# Personality, Mood, and Behavioral Changes

Personality and mood changes in Alzheimer's are more than brain damage. The feeling that your memory is slipping sets off alarm bells in the protective mechanisms of your body. Those alarm bells cause you to worry. That stress can actually cause release of stress hormones that can then cause inflammation, even in the brain, and make your symptoms seem worse.

The list of behaviors that are present in Alzheimer's are long and varied, and include:

- Forgetfulness
- Frustration
- Irritability
- Anxiety
- Depression
- Confusion and mood swings
- Agitation
- Compulsive and ritualistic behavior
- Restlessness
- Delusions
- Psychosis
- Hallucinations

## Forgetfulness and Frustration

Forgetfulness and frustration typically manifest in Stage 2. Memory loss is the first symptom that you get with Alzheimer's. As memory loss increases, so does frustration.

Frustration is not necessarily a behavior; it's more a reaction to what's going on, and it completely describes how you are feeling in the early stages of Alzheimer's.

There are some basic things you can do to help relieve some of your frustration. You're already making notes to yourself, but here are some more tips.

- Exercise your brain cells. Start doing crossword puzzles, join a reading club, and read more "intellectual" books.
- Turn on your computer's memory alert function to remind you of things to do.
- Use brightly colored Post-Its to remind you of things.
- Read books on how to improve your memory.
- Cut down on alcohol, sugar, aspartame sweetener, and MSG. They all interfere with brain function.

## Irritability and Mood Swings

Irritability and mood swings typically manifest themselves in Stages 3 and 4. Frustration leads directly to symptoms of irritability. You get irritable at things and people. You get irritable at people mostly because they complain that you've changed and ask you why you are so upset at seemingly insignificant things. The other side of irritability is that it serves to push people away who might be asking too many questions about what is going on with you. Mostly you are frustrated and mad that you are feeling confused and disoriented and don't know why.

Mood swings are another aspect of Alzheimer's that is hard to ignore. From tears to tantrums in a split second is not unusual. And you don't seem to have any control over these dramatic emotions.

In order to deal with your emotional symptoms, it may be very helpful to seek out a psychologist or psychotherapist.

Support and counseling can help you learn ways to cope with your diagnosis. Counselors also can help sort out the difficult decisions of future living arrangements.

## Confusion and Depression

Confusion and depression typically manifest in Stage 5. Confusion is not really a behavior, but it's how you feel when you can't find something or get lost in a familiar place. One recommendation is to always keep a card with you that says, "I have Alzheimer's, sometimes I get confused, please be patient, here is my address and a number to call for help."

Depression is also a common part of the Alzheimer's picture. You are entitled to feel depressed, but there are ways to cope, people that will support you, and steps you can take to treat depression. Ways of dealing with depression include:

- Talking with a therapist, social worker, or psychotherapist.
- Getting some exercise every day.
- Eating well, getting your sleep, and taking a good multiple vitamin and mineral to make sure you are getting appropriate nutrients.
- Sharing your concerns with your family and planning together for the future.

- Seeing your doctor about taking low levels of appropriate medication for your depression.

## Agitation

The dictionary definition of agitation is nervous anxiety. Agitation is a feeling of not being quite right in your own skin. As the frustration and irritability build, a complex set of behaviors results in agitation. It typically manifests in Stages 5 and 6. Complicating matters even further is the possibility that agitation may be due to coexisting medical conditions and medications that are used in the treatment of Alzheimer's. Physical symptoms of tiredness, lack of sleep, and fatigue can all lead to an increased level of agitation.

Changes in the surrounding environment can also lead to agitation or an increase in symptoms of agitation. Such changes could be moving to a new home or to a nursing home, a change in caregivers, or anything that seems to threaten security and stability.

The obvious recommendations to prevent or treat agitation include trying to keep the living environment as stable and structured as possible.

Agitation can be scary for caregivers as well as for the afflicted individual. Depending on the level of anxiety, agitation can "paralyze" a person and make it difficult for them to go about their daily routine. This makes the role of caregivers even more necessary, yet at the same time, they can become more exhausted by giving constant reassurance to someone who is agitated.

### When to Bring in the Doctor

At the onset of noticeable agitation or if the level of agitation increases drastically, a medical assessment is warranted. Especially if the level of communication is low, someone who is agitated might not know that they have an underlying infection, for example, that could be triggering internal alarms such as fever, pain, dehydration, and general discomfort.

## *Do a Medication and Nutrition Check*

Specific medications may cause agitation; it may happen more often, however, in the case of multiple prescriptions. A pharmacist can often analyze a list of medications and their possible interactions.

Simple dehydration can cause the brain to react in strange ways. Fogginess, dizziness, and lack of concentration are all symptoms of dehydration. The same goes with nutrition; it's crucial to get the right protein, carbohydrates, and fats from the plate into the mouth. Keep a diet log; if you don't, several meals can go by with different caregivers, and your patient hasn't eaten more than a few bites.

### *Treatment for Agitation*

Agitation is treated first with behavioral modification and second with the addition of prescription drugs. In order to apply behavioral modification, you first have to find out what is aggravating the behavior. We must concede that a certain amount of agitation is part of the Alzheimer's picture. But if there is excessive agitation of recent onset, then we must identify the cause and then either eliminate the cause or circumnavigate it.

### How to Avoid and Handle Agitation

Agitation tends to occur episodically. It's important for caregivers to learn how to handle these episodes. Remember, the guiding principle of a caregiver is to offer comfort, dignity, and respect. Your mother, father, or client is agitated for some reason; you may or may not know the reason, but it's important to bring the situation under control.

First of all, let's consider ways to avoid agitation. Eliminate the frustration factor. Organize eating, dressing, and bathing after a rest period and be ready to curtail or modify at the first signs of frustration. Become a master of distraction. Their attention span is very short, and distractions do work. If buttering toast causes frustration, offer a cup of tea. Keep explanations simple. Gently guide activities. Use loving and kind words and gestures. Keep the exit doors locked to prevent wandering. Try to avoid the use of restraints, which causes more agitation.

### How to Divert an Episode of Agitation

It's not always possible to prevent agitation. First, you physically and verbally back away. If arms are flailing or objects are being thrown, don't endanger yourself; don't confront; step back until the moment passes. Be calm and reassuring; when you speak, offer reassurances, apologies, and safety.

Use what you know about your Alzheimer's patient to offer them something they usually see as positive. Of course you must always be aware that there could be an injury, a need to use the bathroom, a need for more light, a hunger, a thirst, or just fatigue. Assess whether a change of scenery or shutting off all stimulation would be appropriate.

### It's Time for Medications

If you've stabilized the home environment and are using behavioral modification, but the level of agitation is escalating, your next step is to turn to medication. Especially when medications become part of the treatment program, an accurate way of monitoring improvement and side effects must be employed. Sometimes, if side effects occur, you can't really tell if they are due to the drug or part of the complex of Alzheimer's symptoms. Make a list of current symptoms before starting any medications and bring this to the doctor.

> The rules in implementing medication are universal, but even more important in Alzheimer's patients. Only start one medication at a time; begin with the lowest dose possible; chart any change in symptoms; and chart any side effects.

## Compulsive Behavior and Restlessness

Humans, in an attempt to influence their fate, will often develop a set of ritual behaviors. Some Alzheimer's sufferers shout out profane words in what appears to be a compulsive way. It's a form of trying to get control of a seemingly uncontrollable situation. Other compulsive behaviors include dry-washing the hands or rubbing parts of the body.

Restlessness is a form of burning off energy that builds up due to frustration and agitation. It can take the form of constant pacing back and forth or checking to see if the stove is off or the doors are locked.

These behaviors are in the later stages of Alzheimer's, and they are very difficult for caregivers to deal with. If you attempt to stop a compulsive or ritualistic behavior, you can cause a considerable amount of distress and agitation in the Alzheimer's sufferer. The most appropriate response is to try to offer a distracting activity, but if that doesn't work, just allow the behavior until they have no more energy for it.

## Severe Mood Swings, Aggressiveness, and Combativeness

Alzheimer's treatment programs call this set of behaviors the "challenging" ones. That's putting a positive spin on behavior that to the outside observer seems to be intent on driving you, the caregiver, crazy.

**How do I justify my feelings of frustration directed at my loved one or patient?**

The tension and frustration you feel as a caregiver is absolutely normal. The main thing to remember is not to take it personally. The behavior you are witnessing has nothing to do with you and everything to do with the person you are caring for.

Repetition of words, although not an aggressive activity, can be very annoying. One way of dealing with this behavior is to say your own repetitive mantra, "this is the disease talking, this is the disease talking." It helps you remember that all these symptoms are, indeed, the result of Alzheimer's.

### Assessing the Cause

As with the other behaviors mentioned, it's time to assess what is causing the mood swings, aggressiveness, and combativeness. The reasons could be so varied that you need a checklist. After a while, the checklist may become automatic and you can, almost intuitively, know what's causing the outrageous behavior.

The reason can range from a new person becoming involved with the patient's care to side effects of medications. They could suddenly be unable to do tasks or activities that they were once able to do and become agitated, or are no longer able to communicate their desires or needs.

### Responding to Challenging Behaviors

How to respond to the challenging behaviors is much like responding to agitation and irritability, but there is a heightened level of intensity and even a feeling of danger that as a caregiver you can't help but feel. But this behavior is occurring in someone who may be your mother or father or a client, and who has no intentions of harming you.

First, become very calm and centered, take deep breaths, and relax. Sometimes your calmness actually rubs off, just as an angry tone or impatience will also be felt. Be very patient and realize you are doing exactly what you should be doing by being very quiet. In our very busy and stressed-out lives, we think we always have to be doing something, and there is no question that there is a lot to do when you are a caregiver for someone with Alzheimer's. But at this moment, you want to stop time and just be.

### Don't Argue

This is the worst time to argue or try to make your mother, father, or client do something they don't want to do. That is often the reason they start to fight you. If they ask or motion to do something else, be flexible and go with their wishes.

As in dealing with agitation, after the dust settles, do a retrospective assessment and try to find the possible cause of the escalation in behavior. Afterward, chart the behavior and make notes about corresponding events and try to understand the pattern of behavior leading up to the event. Above all, seek support and guidance from the doctor or local support groups on coping skills.

## Paranoia, Delusions, and Hallucinations

Paranoia, delusions, and hallucinations are the hallmark symptoms of the final stages of Alzheimer's. Individuals experience symptoms of paranoia during which they really believe someone is breaking into the house, or someone is trying to poison them. Paranoia is an extreme and unreasonable suspicion of other people and their motives. Reassurance is the best way to deal with paranoia.

Delusions can range from patients believing they are being held hostage to being a member of a royal family. In order to deal with delusions, you don't want to enter into the delusion, but you nod and listen and never contradict what the Alzheimer's patient says.

Hallucinations are due to false perceptions; patients may imagine that there are people or things in the room that are not really there. The patient may also experience an auditory hallucination. Sensory hallucinations of touch, taste, and smell can occur when the patient feels something touching or crawling on them, tastes something in their food that isn't there, or smells something. Often the taste and smell hallucinations turn into paranoia about being poisoned or gassed. These are very frightening occurrences.

### Dealing with Hallucinations

Constant reassurance is the best way of dealing with paranoia; hallucinations, however, can be much more difficult to contain. Nodding and agreeing is the best approach. You don't want to start telling them that yes, you see their hallucination, because you can't. But you don't want to deny what they are seeing, either. That will only cause more agitation.

Now is the time to make sure your patient's eyes and ears are functioning optimally. Poor eyesight can make shadows appear real, and poor hearing can turn normal sounds into mumbles.

If hallucinations become constant, it's time to check with the doctor. They may be a result of medication side effects or some acute physical problem not related to Alzheimer's. Even simple dehydration can cause brain irritation that can worsen Alzheimer's symptoms.

All the advice for agitation and challenging behaviors applies here as well. Be calm; be centered; be reassuring; and be supportive. Be ready to talk about your patient's experience if he or she wants to. Distraction works for hallucinations as well as other symptoms of Alzheimer's.

When you see the telltale signs of eyes focusing on nothing, an ear cocked when there is no sound, or hands flicking off imaginary bugs, just put a reassuring hand on the patient's shoulder, and they may snap out of their hallucination when they look at you. Increasing the lighting can help remove shadows or reflections. Putting on some gentle music or moving to another room can also banish hallucinations. One common recommendation is to remove or cover mirrors, because at this stage, your patient may see a stranger looking back at them.

# Chapter 6

# Medical Treatment for Alzheimer's

As we further our understanding of what causes damage to the brain and consequent symptoms, we learn how to prevent and delay the process. The current focus of treatment is on the alleviation of symptoms and on early diagnosis of Alzheimer's. Many of the newer drugs available can help people improve their mental symptoms for months to years, increasing the chances of finding a cure in time to help them.

## Medical Treatment Strategies

There are three aspects of Alzheimer's disease that can be treated with medications: cognitive symptoms (memory, thinking, and perception), behavioral symptoms (agitation, anxiety, and irritability), and insomnia.

It is important, however, to begin with only one medication at a time, use the lowest dose possible to achieve the most benefit, and chart any and all changes in symptoms. These drugs must be used with caution, and caregivers need to be aware of these possible side effects.

The U.S. Food and Drug Administration (FDA) has approved two classes of drugs to treat cognitive symptoms of Alzheimer's disease: cholinesterase inhibitors and NMDA(N-methyl-D-aspartate) receptor antagonists, also called glutamate blockers. To date, five drugs are FDA approved for use in treating Alzheimer's cognitive symptoms. (Many more are in the research pipeline.) The following four are from the class of drugs called cholinesterase inhibitors:

1. Cognex (THA)
2. Aricept

3. Reminyl
4. Exelon

## Cholinesterase Inhibitors

Cholinesterase inhibitors act to prevent breakdown of a very important neurotransmitter called acetylcholine. Acetylcholine is found in the brain and spinal cord and in nerve/muscle junctions. It is made from acetyl CoA and choline. After acetylcholine is produced, it normally transmits a message and is then broken down, by a special enzyme called cholinesterase, back to its original constituents—acetyl CoA and choline.

> Cholinesterase inhibitor drugs prevent the breakdown of acetylcholine, thus allowing it to build up, and make more acetylcholine available in the brain to carry messages between the brain cells.

Research shows that cholinesterase inhibitors that act on the brain increase cerebral blood flow when measured by SPECT scans. The increased blood flow is in brain regions affected by

Alzheimer's disease. They only work, however, in the mild to moderate stages of Alzheimer's disease because functioning nerve cells are necessary to make acetylcholine in the first place.

### Cognex—The First Alzheimer's Drug

Cognex was the first Alzheimer's drug approved by the FDA (1993). It has a long and unpronounceable scientific name, Tetrahydroaminoacridine; the short form is THA, and the drug name is Cognex. It's a "crossover" drug. It's a cholinesterase inhibitor, but it also has beneficial effects on behavior.

In most patients who took Cognex, doctors found moderate improvement in cognitive symptoms with no change in the progression of the disease. It also has a dramatic effect on the behavior of an Alzheimer's sufferer. Most notable is a decrease in symptoms such as apathy, irritability, and agitation.

Fifty percent of all people who take Cognex have a rise in liver enzymes after a month or six weeks on the drug. For this reason it is rarely prescribed.

Drug interactions can occur with other medicines that increase acetylcholine activity. These include medicines for myasthenia gravis, other Alzheimer's medicines and medicines for urinary retention.

### *Aricept*

Aricept, approved in 1996, was designed to be a substitute for Cognex and its toxic liver effects. Its generic name is donepezil. It is specifically intended for people with mild to moderate Alzheimer's disease, but it won't help everybody, and it is not a cure. It does one of four things: It can do nothing; it may cause symptoms to improve; it may halt the progression of symptoms; or it could cause side effects.

In one study, compared to the effects of a placebo, 50 percent of the placebo group got worse, which is the normal course of events. But only about 33 percent of those on Aricept got worse. Those people on Aricept were twice as likely to show some improvement in thinking, understanding, problem solving, and overall symptoms. In those patients that improved, if they stopped Aricept after two years, it took another six months for Alzheimer's symptoms to become worse.

Aricept comes in two strengths, 5 milligrams and 10 milligrams, to be taken once a day in the evening. It is a good idea to start on the lower dose to lessen any side effects. It does have side effects of diarrhea, nausea, vomiting, muscle cramps, insomnia, loss of appetite, and fatigue; they mostly occur at the beginning of treatment and usually subside. Aricept could possibly worsen the symptoms of stomach ulcers, asthma, and some heart diseases.

Aricept may interact with some antidepressants, anesthetics, antihistamines, and some painkillers. Your doctor or pharmacist should be aware of all your medications.

### Reminyl

Reminyl was approved for the treatment of mild to moderate Alzheimer's in 2000. Its generic name is galantamine. It has much the same indications and moderately successful effects as

Aricept, as it is also a cholinesterase inhibitor. Large placebo-controlled, double-blind studies on about 3,000 patients over six months have been done on Reminyl. In one study, on an Alzheimer's scoring system, there was no change in score; in another study, one-third of patients improved their score by four points. The usual annual increase in symptoms is between five and eleven points. 15 percent of people taking the placebo, however, also improved by the same amount in exactly the same way.

Reminyl treats cognitive symptoms, but it is also beneficial for behavioral symptoms such as anxiety, hallucinations, and wandering. In one five-month study, patients' behavioral symptoms as well as activities of daily living did not worsen, whereas those on placebo worsened significantly.

Reminyl comes in 4 milligram, 8 milligram, and 12 milligram tablets. The initial dosage is 4 milligrams twice per day. After one month, the dose may be increased.

The most common side effects are nausea and vomiting, which usually go away with time. Other less common side effects may occur. Rarely, trembling, a slow heartbeat, or fainting may occur.

Drug interactions with Reminyl come mainly from Parkinson's drugs, drugs that treat diarrhea and asthma, as well as heart drugs. A lower dose of Reminyl may be necessary if you are taking antidepressants or an HIV drug. Reminyl should not be taken if you have severe liver and/or kidney disease. Your doctor will watch you closely if you have acute abdominal pain, asthma, epilepsy, heart disease, liver or kidney problems, ulcers, urinary retention, an allergy to the pill's lactose or yellow dye coating, or have had recent surgery.

## Exelon

Exelon is the brand name for rivastigmine, a cholinesterase inhibitor approved by the FDA in 2000 for mild to moderately severe Alzheimer's disease. By the time it reached the market, about 5,200 people had been treated. Exelon increases the level of acetylcholine in the brain to improve thinking, learning, memory, and the symptoms of dementia and daily functioning in Alzheimer's disease.

A dosage of 1.5 milligrams of Exelon is taken twice daily in capsule form with meals. The maximum dose is 6 milligrams twice daily. The main side effects may include nausea, vomiting, abdominal pain, and loss of appetite, which lessen as your system gets used to the drug. Other less common side effects may occur.

Exelon should be used with caution in those with asthma, chronic obstructive pulmonary disease, epilepsy, heart rhythm problems, decreased kidney function, Parkinson's disease, peptic ulcer, and sick sinus syndrome.

## Medications for Agitation

There really isn't a specific "agitation" medication. Since agitation in Alzheimer's is a combination of anxiety, depression, and irritability, there are a variety of medications that might prove useful. Antidepressant medications that can help the depression and irritability include Celexa, Paxil, Prozac, and Zoloft. Shorter acting drugs that are used for the treatment of anxiety, restlessness, verbal aggression, and resistant behavior include anxiolytics such as Ativan and Serax.

If the anti-anxiety and antidepressant drugs don't work or if the patient is within the worsening stages of agitation, stronger medications called antipsychotics are used. For these patients, agitation is accompanied by delusions, hallucinations, aggressive behavior, hostility, and a total lack of cooperation. The names of these medications are Zyprexa and Risperdal.

Additional drugs that treat agitation include anticonvulsants such as Tegretol; these drugs also treat mood swings. Depakote has been used to partially treat hostility and aggression.

### Sleeping Medications

Sleeping medications are called sedatives. They slow down a person's functioning on all levels, not just the nervous system. They may cause drowsiness, but they also cause a lot of other side effects. They can cause incontinence, imbalance, falling, and increased agitation.

At first you might think the side effects of these drugs are symptoms of worsening Alzheimer's. Stopping the medication, however, will cause a reversal of symptoms. If these drugs are used, they must be used very cautiously with awareness of their potential side effects.

## Clinical Trials

It is possible that you or your loved one may be asked to participate in a clinical trial. It seems like every month, drug companies are announcing a new Alzheimer's drug that they feel will be the answer. All these drugs must eventually be tested on Alzheimer's patients, and you may be one of them. You and your family may even want to be proactive about entering a clinical trial so you can be in on the latest developments from pharmaceutical companies.

**How do I get involved in a clinical trial?**

The Alzheimer's Association and many other Alzheimer's organizations and hospitals have specific information about clinical trials.

You will want to know what they are, how they work, who gets to participate, and the risks and benefits; you will also need help with making a decision about entering a trial.

## What Is a Clinical Trial?

Briefly, a clinical trial is a necessary part of drug research to find out if a new drug is safe and effective in a human population. By the time a drug gets to the human trial stage, it has been proven safe in animals. A clinical trial protocol defines who can participate in a study and all the tests, procedures, medications, and dosages that are prescribed, as well as the duration of the study. Drug companies usually pay for clinical trials, and researchers or doctors in hospitals or universities run the trials.

The best part of a clinical trial is that frequent appointments are made for patients to see the research staff in order to monitor symptoms, both good and bad. The worst part is that you may or may not get the real drug. If the trial is a placebo-control, you may get the placebo (the inactive pill).

## The Institutional Review Board

An Institutional Review Board (IRB), usually in a hospital or university, is set up to oversee and monitor every clinical trial in the United States.

The IRB members are independent physicians, statisticians, and community advocates who ensure that a clinical trial is ethical and the participants' rights are protected. The IRB ensures that the risks of a particular study are as low as possible and that the benefits outweigh the risks.

### Informed Consent

Most of us are familiar with signing an informed consent paper for surgery. It's the same with a clinical trial. Researchers are obliged to inform you of all the important aspects of the research trial, including the type of drug or treatment, the side effects, the expected benefits, whether similar treatments are available, and your right to leave the trial at any time. After you and your family are clear on all aspects of the trial, you will be asked to sign an informed consent.

## Regular Checkups with Your Doctor

It's important to have regular checkups with your doctor to monitor your condition and your response to any medications you may be on. Your doctor will have done what's called a baseline assessment, using specific tests, during your initial visits for Alzheimer's. This assessment is kept on record, and at all other visits, the tests are repeated and compared to the first. It's important to have this baseline to know how you felt and what symptoms you had when you were first diagnosed and also to help evaluate medications.

The most common medical test is the Mini-Mental State Examination (MMSE) given by a doctor. Another test is a questionnaire called the Physical Self-Maintenance Scale (PSMS), which can be filled out by a caregiver. Both of them together help establish baseline memory, thinking, language, and functional ability. Behavioral symptoms, such as agitation, psychosis, anxiety, and depression, are also on record as part of the baseline assessment.

### Ongoing Evaluation

Your doctor will usually see you every three to six months after your initial diagnosis, and every three months if you have started any medication. When you are stabilized on the medication, the visits are usually every six months.

Your doctor will perform the MMSE, PSMS, and a behavioral assessment at each visit to follow any change in your symptoms. If you begin experiencing more severe symptoms like depression, agitation, hallucinations, or delirium, you may be started on a different medication and see your doctor more often. If you develop other conditions or symptoms, not necessarily associated with Alzheimer's, regular visits with your doctor will help monitor these as well.

### Treatment Evaluation

When your doctor evaluates your response to medication, it is mainly to see if there is stabilization of your condition. Sometimes dramatic improvements do take place but not as often as we would wish. If a sharp decline is noted after initiating a new medicine, your doctor may ask you and your caregiver to stop the medication or slowly wean off it.

Your doctor will also make sure you and your caregiver understand that there is, as yet, no cure for Alzheimer's; the current medications are limited and cannot stop or reverse the natural progression of the disease.

The medications currently available do allow a longer period of independence and may help delay the need for a nursing home or other institutionalized care.

### Caregiving at Your Appointments

Your caregiver, for many reasons, should accompany you to every doctor's appointment. You may need assistance getting to the appointment and undressing and dressing for your physical exam. Your caregiver can also help recount your symptoms since your last visit, any major life changes (such as a move or a hospitalization), and what medications you are taking. Your caregiver will bring your medications to the appointment.

## *Assessment Tools*

You or your family and caregivers may want to know what assessment tools are used in Alzheimer's. There are four categories.

1. **Cognitive Assessments**, which measure thinking, learning, and memory.

    - Alzheimer's Disease Assessment Scale, cognitive subsection (ADAS-cog)
    - Blessed Information-Memory-Concentration Test (BIMC)
    - Clinical Dementia Rating Scale (CDR)
    - Mini-Mental State Examination (MMSE)

2. **Functional Assessments**, which measure activities of daily living and ability to function on a daily basis.

    - Functional Assessment Questionnaire (FAQ)
    - Instrumental Activities of Daily Living (IADL)
    - Physical Self-Maintenance Scale (PSMS)
    - Progressive Deterioration Scale (PDS)

3. **Global Assessments**, which assess both cognitive symptoms and functional symptoms.

  - Clinical Global Impression of Change (CGIC)
  - Clinical Interview-Based Impression (CIBI)
  - Global Deterioration Scale (GDS)

4. **Caregiver-Based Assessments.**

  - Behavioral Pathology in Alzheimer's Disease Rating Scale (BEHAVE-AD)
  - Neuropsychiatric Inventory (NPI)

# Chapter 7

# Caregivers Coping and Caring

When it comes to Alzheimer's, we all must learn coping skills to deal with the disease. If you have been diagnosed with Alzheimer's, you've been told there is no cure. You must learn to cope with the finality of that statement and calmly come to peace with it. Your caregivers also learn to cope; they learn how to support you as they render care, especially if they put themselves in your place.

## The Caregiver's Role

Caregiver status is not as valued as it should be, but it is slowly becoming recognized. There is the observation that caregiving is meeting a deep need in our society at great emotional, physical, mental, and financial costs to the caregiver. There is also the recognition that caregiving can be taught, and by so doing, caregivers can carry out their role a little more easily with the right tools and the right support.

### The Gift of Caring

Caregiving has a major focus on helping people. What many find out is that by caring for and helping others, you nourish your own soul. Giving the gift of caring to another actually allows you to reap many intangible rewards.

Many caregivers say they feel honored to participate in the deep intimacy of someone else's life. The skills learned in caring for someone with Alzheimer's are invaluable for any life challenge.

## How to Be a Good Communicator

As a caregiver, you may take a special course in caregiving or just depend on your common sense and love to see you through. Please know, however, that there is a tremendous support system and network for you to tap into: support groups, books, articles, online support, and much more.

Communication with an Alzheimer's sufferer means you have to get them to focus on you. Get rid of distractions first. We often spend our day at home with a TV or radio on in the background and tune it out. But someone with Alzheimer's may find such things very distracting when you are trying to talk with them.

Don't talk from across the room; get close enough to have eye contact in order to get and keep their attention. Don't give long-winded explanations of what you want to do; they may forget the first of it by the time you finish.

Just simply state what you want. Let's go for a walk. Let's brush your hair. Say sentences that ask for agreement rather than offering a choice, which may be confusing. And try not to sound reprimanding when you tell them not to do things. You must not speak down to them; just speak clearly and slowly with a lot of repetition.

### Communication Tools: The Do's

One special Web site, Health and Age (*www .healthandage.com*), features wonderful articles that give useful advice on many aspects of caring for Alzheimer's. A particularly helpful article, which was modified from a publication by the Alzheimer's Association, called "How to Talk to Someone with Alzheimer's," by Dr. Robert Griffith, helps us with the very first step of how to communicate.

In your relationship with an Alzheimer's patient, here are the tools you can apply to make your communication meaningful. Dr. Griffith says talking with someone with Alzheimer's is a skill that requires time and patience, but it all boils down to being a good listener. Dr. Griffith recommends several helpful do's:

- Approach from the front, make eye contact, and say your name if you aren't recognized.
- Speak slowly, calmly, and use a friendly facial expression.
- Use short, simple, and familiar words.
- Show that you are listening and trying to understand what is being said.
- Be careful not to interrupt; avoid arguing and criticizing.
- Ask one question at a time, and allow time for a reply.
- Make positive suggestions (e.g., "Let's go into the garden") rather than negative ones (e.g., "Don't go in there").
- Identify others by name, rather than using pronouns (she, he, etc.).
- Make suggestions if the person has trouble choosing.
- Empathize; have patience and understanding. Touch or hug, if it helps.

### Communication Tools: The Don'ts

If your Alzheimer's patient is caught in a memory loop about their past, don't ask questions that they might not be able to answer. Instead, offer praise and support for whatever they have done in their life. The following are important don'ts:

- Don't talk about the person as if he or she weren't there.
- Don't confront or correct, if it can be avoided.
- Don't treat the person as a child, but as an adult.

### Continuing the Conversation

Dr. Griffith wrote an update on his former paper about how to talk with someone with Alzheimer's; he gives more advice for the more serious or more challenging cases:

- Take your time and look for a response to your voice. A hearing disability may make it even harder for someone to communicate.
- When the person replies, show that you are listening and trying to understand.
- Give plenty of encouragement and reassurance—touching or hugging may help.

- Allow time for the reply—don't interrupt, argue, or criticize. Remember, you will never win an argument with an Alzheimer's person.
- If the person seems stuck for a word, you can offer a guess, but act like you have all the time in the world.
- If you aren't quite sure you understood what was said, repeat it back and ask if you've got it right.
- Try to understand the person's feelings and emotions, which may be hidden behind the words. You can ask whether the person is feeling angry or frustrated about a particular situation.
- Make allowances for digressions (reminiscences, backtracking, repetitions, etc.). However, if necessary, prompt the person gently, so they can get back on track.
- Choose a quiet time and place for your discussion, so that both of you are free from interruptions and distractions.
- Be aware that the person may want to point or gesture, if at a loss for words.

### Communicating with Visitors

Nonverbal communication such as shaking hands is such a learned behavior that you can include the Alzheimer's patient in such a greeting; even if they don't remember the visitor's name, they can nod and shake hands. A friendly smile and "hello" with an outstretched hand will often elicit a handshake and a "thank you, just fine."

**How can I make it less embarrassing for a person with Alzheimer's when they don't remember who someone is?**

You can make it much easier by introducing the visitor by name and give a little description so that the Alzheimer's patient can give a response.

Doing this will include them in the conversation and relieve the awkwardness and embarrassment of not remembering the visitor's name.

## Caregiver Behavior Skills

There is a set of skills that may or may not come naturally to a caregiver, but from whatever place you start on your caregiving journey, you can certainly learn from others that have been there, and you will definitely learn from your Alzheimer's patient as well. Let's take a look at the various skills a caregiver needs to have in his or her arsenal.

### Detachment

Learning to detach goes under the heading of "don't take it personally; don't react." Don't think that your Alzheimer's patient means disrespect or anger, or that his or her irritability is directed at you personally. It's usually the disease talking.

Misunderstanding, frustration, and confusion make many people with Alzheimer's very irritable. The usual human reaction to frustration is to blame someone else. And you, as the caregiver, are often that someone. Knowing that it's the disease talking can help you step back.

That being said, there are ornery people in the world, and Alzheimer's isn't going to make that go away; that behavior might get worse. In this case, you may need to learn to "turn the other cheek."

### Patience

Some Alzheimer's patients become meek and very needy. They need constant reassurance and attention. This type of behavior can also be very frustrating, and this is where even more patience is necessary. Patience is important in every facet of Alzheimer's caregiving. Your patient is going to be very slow about every activity, and you must be willing to go slowly, too. Deep breathing, slow counting, and reciting poetry are all useful ways of developing patience and learning to slow down your normal pace. Especially if you work at another job during the day and are a caregiver at night, you need to switch off the fast-paced work mode and get into caregiver mode.

## *Compassion and Empathy*

When laypeople go to a religious retreat to gain greater spiritual depth and wisdom, they may be given the wise counsel to seek spirituality by unselfishly helping others. Some call it unconditional love. You feel it when you expect nothing back from the person you are caring for. By tapping into this unconditional love, you will feel greater empathy and compassion for your Alzheimer's patient and a very strong connection to your spirituality.

After all, when it all comes down to the question of life and death, you are ready to ask the important questions. What would I consider the most important thing in my life if I know I am going to die tomorrow? Most people answer that their family, friends, and loved ones are the most important thing. Material goods and societal accomplishments pale in comparison to a meaningful relationship with other human beings.

## Scheduling Care at Home

Most people with Alzheimer's are taken care of at home by family and friends. The decision is often made immediately to have their loved one be cared for at home as long as possible. The family doesn't want to "abandon" their mother or father to an institution. There is a perception that care in nursing homes is not up to par, and they are often more than the family can afford.

> Care at home means you need to create a schedule where four or five team members each cover a day and a half. Or, each team member may take one week on duty and rotate every month.

Either way, it usually means that part of the team is working full-time and will have to make adjustments to their schedules.

If you are a professional, you may be able to schedule your appointments to allow time off to do "your shift." If you aren't in control of your schedule, you may find it more difficult to find time for your shift. That's when sick days, vacation days, weekends, and holidays all go into the caregiving pot. For all concerned, caregiving either means a loss of income or much more stress; often it is both.

## Care for the Caregiver

Taking care of someone who has Alzheimer's disease can be exhausting, frustrating, and overwhelming. Detachment is an easy word to say but very difficult to perform. Patience, compassion, and empathy also take their toll. Taking care of a loved one is hard work. You are responsible for their every need, but who's taking care of you?

### *Caregiver's Bill of Rights*

As a caregiver for an Alzheimer's patient, you are often expected to be superhuman. The American Health Assistance Foundation understands the problems of caregiving, and through the Alzheimer's Family Relief Program, they make sure people know their rights. One of the first rights is the right to be human, to have human emotions and human needs.

The Caregiver's Bill of Rights may seem like common sense, but it's necessary to keep the advice it gives utmost in your mind so you can maintain your mental and physical balance for yourself and your loved one. The Bill of Rights states that it's all right to have normal human emotions, but then make sure you turn that emotion into something more positive. It's okay to:

**Be angry.** Work off this energy physically; take a walk, clean closets, talk it over with someone.

**Be frustrated.** Count to ten and stop doing what is making you frustrated and do something else.

**Taketime alone.** Find a few minutes or hours to be alone.

**Ask for help.** Canvas family, friends, and local Alzheimer's support groups for support.

**Trust your judgment.** Trust that you are doing the best you can and realize you can't do more than that.

**Recognize your limits.** It's of no use to you or your Alzheimer's patient to stretch yourself to your limit. You are a valuable person. Take care of yourself, too!

**Make mistakes.** We learn through our mistakes. No one is perfect.

**Grieve.** It's okay and perfectly normal to be going through a grief response for the loss of the way things were.

**Laugh and love.** Laughter and love heal all wounds.

**Hope.** Each new day may be better, may be easier, and a cure may be found.

### Guilt

You may not know it, but you may be feeling guilty about your loved one's situation. You consciously or unconsciously may say, "Why should I feel fine if my loved one isn't?" And psychologically, people sometimes punish themselves when their loved one is ill. In some cultures, cutting off a finger when someone dies is normal. We don't go quite that far, but the tendency is there to try to take some of their burden by becoming ill ourselves. We need to guard against this.

We also feel guilty if we find ourselves being happy or excited about something, and then feel like we are betraying our loved one and their suffering. But they wouldn't want your life to end because they are ill. We need to keep our perspective of life and death and realize that by our suffering, we aren't making their suffering less. If we can maintain a cheerful outlook and give a genuine smile, we can lift the spirits of our Alzheimer's sufferer and lift our own spirits as well.

### The Caregiver Stress Test

This test is in a book called the *Caregiver's Handbook*, edited by Robert Torres-Stanovick and published by the San Diego County Mental Health Services in 1990. Caregivers are instructed to answer the following questions using the most appropriate word(s): Seldom, Sometimes, Often, Usually True, Always True.

1. I find I can't get enough rest.
2. I don't have enough time for myself.
3. I don't have time to be with other family members besides the person I care for.
4. I feel guilty about my situation.
5. I don't get out much anymore.

6. I have conflict with the person I care for.
7. I have conflict with other family members.
8. I cry every day.
9. I worry about having enough money to make ends meet.
10. I don't feel I have enough knowledge or experience to give care as well as I'd like.
11. My own health is not good.

Caregivers are further instructed that if they respond with "Usually True" or "Always True" in one or more of these areas, it may be time to begin looking for help with caring for the Alzheimer's patient and help in taking care of him or herself.

# Chapter 8

# Caregiving at Home

Creating a safe and comfortable home environment for your Alzheimer's patient is doable, but it's important to enlist your family and friends. You'll have to tackle every room in the house and make sure it is safe for someone with Alzheimer's. It is a difficult process, time consuming, and tedious, but with the following plan in hand, it will make life much easier for everyone. First let's see who's going to be in charge.

## Caring for Your Spouse

When your spouse receives a diagnosis of Alzheimer's, you are probably living independently in your house or apartment, in which case the task of caregiving falls on your shoulders. If the disease is in the early stages, then it's a matter of giving love and support, accompanying your spouse to doctor's appointments, meeting with the family, and eventually making appointments with your spouse's employer, your lawyer, and your financial advisor.

Then you have to take stock of the home environment and see how to make things safe as your spouse's memory becomes more impaired.

If you don't have family nearby to help, there are numerous organizations that can lend a hand. It's a matter of reaching out and asking for help. Nobody caring for someone with Alzheimer's should feel that they are alone.

When the task of caring for your spouse becomes too great, then you must rely on your family's support. If you don't have family, again, there are many agencies, foundations, and associations dedicated to helping those with Alzheimer's.

## Family Choices

As a family, when you begin to see a problem with your relative, there is the conscious or unconscious shuffling about to see who is going to take charge of the situation. Temporary, and sometimes ineffectual, measures are often taken that make you feel better but don't really improve the situation. For example, you may feel the need to install safety locks or alarm systems, thinking that your elderly relative, who lives alone, needs to be protected. That can backfire because they can't remember the numbers for the alarm or figure out how to use the lock because their short-term memory is impaired.

Often, the next step is to find a housekeeper or caregiver to stay with your relative if that can be afforded. If not, then there is the inevitable move into one of your homes. Hopefully, this is decided in a family meeting where everyone agrees who should be the primary caregiver and what support the rest of the family members are offering.

## Sibling Involvement

Even at the best of times, not all siblings get along. There is considerable stress involved with caregiving, and it's not unusual for tensions to become even more strained. It's important in communicating with your siblings to keep uppermost in your minds that it's not about you and not about them; it's about your parent. Regular meetings, in person or over the telephone, are important to keep open the lines of communication.

You may find that one of your siblings is more concerned about their needs than your parent's and draws away from involvement. If they are in poor health and under considerable stress, they may not be able to physically lend a hand. You can, however, keep them in the information loop and ask if they can help financially.

At some point, the family may want to sit with a trained Alzheimer's counselor to help with family communication and to help set priorities. Most families are not trained in either caregiving or communication, so it's an opportunity to learn how to deal with problems head-on, by keeping a level head, reining in your emotions, and communicating openly and honestly. Many issues have to be dealt with, and each one may need to be negotiated to achieve a consensus. Again, uppermost in your minds should be the comfort of your relative.

## When the Nuclear Family Is Involved

It appears that many nuclear families have no choice but to get involved. In a 1998 report called "Who Cares," the Alzheimer's Association and the National Alliance for Caregiving found that at least one in three families caring for Alzheimer's sufferers also cared for children under the age of eighteen.

We all know what happens if there are two or more children in the house—sibling rivalry. And with every new addition to the home, whether a child or an aging grandparent, there is a major shift in family dynamics. People who feel love and care is finite will be afraid that they won't get as much love and attention. Well, love isn't finite; it's boundless, but there will definitely be less time spent on other family members if the major caregiver is also taking care of someone with Alzheimer's.

### Children's Concerns

Children living with an Alzheimer's patient can feel angry, jealous, sad, and even guilty, wondering, "Is Grandma crazy? Can I get Alzheimer's, or will my mom and dad get it?"

Children may display behavior such as withdrawing from the loved one, becoming impatient with the person, doing poorly in school, and complaining of headaches, stomachaches, or other minor ailments. (This information comes from *www.mayoclinic.com* and *wcnn.com*.

Caring for an Alzheimer's patient at home is even harder with very young children who don't know what Alzheimer's disease is and just think Granddad is acting weird or scary. If you are the primary caregiver and a mother as well, your children may be acting out in an attempt to get your attention. For some kids, negative attention is better than no attention, and acting out may be the only way they know how to get it.

### Getting the Children Involved

To prevent the almost inevitable clash when dealing with the demands of caring for your relative, start having weekly family meetings and get everyone involved with the project of helping. Give the meetings a special name that everyone agrees on such as Granddad's Team Meeting, or Grandma's Club. In the meetings, ask everyone, even young children, for their advice. This approach can turn up incredibly helpful suggestions and elicit children's support. Being asked gives children a real "buy in" to the new situation.

Instead of trying to protect children from what you see as a very difficult situation, get them involved. Give young children chores such as giving five hugs a day to you and, if they feel comfortable, to their grandparent. If possible, try to "reframe" the task of helping your loved one as an adventure and not a burden. Kids can appreciate an adventure much more than a burden.

Caregiver respite services, where a volunteer comes to the home once or twice a week for four hours or so, can give the family time for a much-needed outing and quality time together. You also need to build time together into your daily schedule. Maybe it's over breakfast or dinner or some other convenient time when everyone is together and your relative is sleeping. It's a time to catch up with what's happening at school or what's happening at your spouse's workplace.

## Safeguarding Your Loved One

Considering all the ways an Alzheimer's patient can get into trouble, you'll find that protecting them is very much like protecting a child. Think of them wandering off unattended, grabbing a sharp knife by the blade, dropping an electric shaver in a sink of water or a full tub, or tripping on a loose carpet. You can protect them from all these things by following certain commonsense guidelines.

*In case of wandering:*

- Have your Alzheimer's relative wear an ID bracelet so rescuers, local police, medical staff, and others are alerted to his or her condition in the event of an emergency.
- Keep a recent photo and, better still, a video of your patient available.
- Use iron-on labels with the Alzheimer's patient's name, address, and phone number in his or her clothing to aid in identification.

*In the home:*

- Purchase rubber-soled shoes or slippers for your loved one to help avoid falls.
- Arrange furniture so he or she can move around easily.
- Eliminate or firmly tape down any scatter rugs, area rugs, or moveable carpets.
- Use nightlights to make finding the bathroom easier at night.
- Remove firearms and weapons from your home.
- Lock up over-the-counter medicines, prescription medicines, and cleaning fluids.

- Keep alcohol in a locked cabinet and away from your relative.
- Use bed rails or place a comforter or pillows on the floor around the bed in case of falling.
- Hide car keys and, if necessary, disconnect the car battery if the patient is not allowed to drive but refuses to stop.
- If the patient hallucinates or is bothered by his or her reflection, cover or remove all mirrors.
- Use a baby sound monitor in his or her room if you are in a different part of the house.
- Do not leave your relative alone in a parked car.
- Use safe plastic fans that won't cut the fingers if poked.
- If necessary, build a wheelchair ramp.

*For the caregiver:*

- Keep a working flashlight by your bed.
- Keep medical records on hand at all times.

## Alzheimer's Safety in the Home

If you can remember a time when you felt spaced out and disoriented, such as after being up all night, or after surgery, or in the middle of a bad flu, you know how unstable you feel; you are constantly apologizing for bumping into things and forgetting things. Well, with Alzheimer's, that seems to be the pervasive feeling. Because of a very short attention span, problems naming and recognizing things, the inability to make decisions, and problems communicating desires, anything can go wrong.

The familiar act of boiling water on the stove can be forgotten as your Alzheimer's relative wanders away on some elusive task. The result is a burned kettle or, even worse, a fire or a severe skin burn when the white hot kettle is not recognized as dangerous.

Candles left burning can be another danger, as can leaving the doors wide open for strangers to come in, or leaving the bathtub filling up with water until the house is flooded.

Supervision is the most important aspect of keeping your Alzheimer's relative safe, but you cannot be there all the time. So, it's important to make sure various rooms have simple safety features that help make your job easier.

### Bathroom Safety

Safety in the bathroom is important for all members of the family but most important for the elderly. When injuries happen in a seemingly safe environment, such as a bathroom, it can serve to greatly erode confidence and can be a major setback even if there is no broken bone.

Starting with the tub, install safety bars on the sides of the tub; place a rubber bath mat or adhesive decals on the floor of the tub or shower; place a bath chair in the tub that is stable and secure; install a soap and shampoo rack on a level where standing and reaching are not required; install a handheld shower nozzle so the shower doesn't beat down on the head; and keep several bath mats on the side of the tub to prevent a severe head injury from an unexpected fall on the edge.

**Is there a way to make the toilet safer for my patient or loved one?**

Install a raised toilet seat with special side rails for holding onto while getting on and off the toilet.

The faucets of the sink may need to be padded to prevent injury from a fall. Wrapping a facecloth around and securing with an elastic band may do the trick. Some people advise using permanent marker to label the taps with red for hot and blue for cold as a reminder. The bathroom medicine cabinet should be locked or else everything should be removed from it.

Lastly, a rubber-backed mat is important to have in the bathroom to prevent slips and falls on a floor made wet by a bath or steam from a bath. Throw out the fluffy bath mat that may trip someone who has a slow, shuffling gait.

### Kitchen Safety

Whether it's a gas range or electric, the stove is the most dangerous appliance in the kitchen.

You can effectively neutralize the danger by removing the stove's knobs. When you want to use the stove, replace them; when you are finished, take the knobs off again and store them in a safe hiding place. While using the stove, if your Alzheimer's patient is in the kitchen, it's best to keep pot handles pointing to the back of the stove so your patient can't accidentally grab or bump them.

Many kitchen fires and house fires start with fat or oil that is left on the stove and forgotten about. It grows hotter, begins to smoke, and eventually bursts into flame, spraying oil and flames around the room. Another kitchen hazard comes from spilling water into a pan of heated oil, causing splashing oil that can catch fire on a gas cooking flame.

Drawers hold potentially lethal knives and scissors, which must be removed and safely stored. Kitchen cabinets under the sink usually contain unsafe cleaning supplies and must be padlocked. Even overhead cabinets can be unsafe; if your Alzheimer's patient tries to get something, cans and/or boxes can fall on his or her head. The kitchen is the place to keep the house fire extinguisher because most fires start in the kitchen. It's also the place for emergency numbers on a magnet pad on the fridge. And finally, mats in the kitchen should be avoided, as they can cause falls from being tripped over or slipped on.

### Door, Window, and Stair Safety

Patient wandering is a common problem for Alzheimer's caregivers to deal with, so doors must be kept locked or equipped with childproof doorknobs. As extra protection you might have to install some sort of alarm or bell system on doors to the outside. There should also be locks on windows and patio doors.

For stair safety, what seems to work for children also works for wandering adults. This includes putting up a gate at the top and bottom of the stairs and locking the bolt. A handrail on the stair is a necessity; if you can put one on either side, so much the better. Bright duct tape across the top and bottom of each step can help to guide an Alzheimer's patient safely up and down stairs.

## *Fire and Electrical Safety*

Fire safety is important because a match can be struck, electrical cords can be tampered with, paper can be stuffed around a radiator, a space heater can be knocked over, or the stove or fireplace can be turned on by someone who doesn't realize what they are doing.

Keeping matches and lighters out of reach, removing electrical wires, covering radiators, using childproof covers on plugs, and not using space heaters are the first steps to preventing a fire.

We already know there should be a fire extinguisher in the kitchen, but if there is more than one floor, each floor should have a fire extinguisher. Smoke detectors should also be installed on each floor and in your relative's bedroom. Fire drills are important so that you know the best ways out in case of a fire.

# Chapter 9

# Choosing Care Outside the Home

As Alzheimer's progresses, it's possible that you will need to have round-the-clock care. Physically, emotionally, and financially, you just may not be able to meet that challenge. And you shouldn't have to. Planning now for long-term care can be a great relief to everyone and relieve your loved one of thinking that they are going to be a burden or wondering how they will spend their last days.

## Adult Day Care

Along the caregiving path, you may have become involved with adult day care, placing your relative in a day care facility that had a specialized dementia-care program, while you worked. You may have home care services, meals on wheels, visiting homemakers, and visiting nurses that help share the burden of care and responsibility. Even coordinating these services calls for planning and organization in your busy day as a caregiver.

The ARCH National Respite Network and Resource Center, funded in part by the U.S. Department of Health and Human Services, produced an important information handout on adult day care in 2002. They call it "One Form of Respite for Older Adults."

Adult day care has grown because of Medicaid waiver programs that find it cost effective to support alternatives to institutional long-term care. Mary Brugger Murphy, director of National Adult Day Services Association (NADSA), reports that "many of the people served by adult day centers would have been institutionalized just ten years ago."

Adult day care centers provide an opportunity for a person with Alzheimer's to socialize with friends while offering respite to their caregiver. Some caregivers, however, have to use adult day care in order to continue to work at their full-time jobs.

Just as they do their children, adult children with an Alzheimer's parent will drop them off at day care and continue on to their job, picking them up after work and taking them home to continue their care.

In an adult day care, participants can also obtain health services and therapeutic services according to their needs. Some adult day care centers have specific services for dementia, which means they can offer activities and exercise that help improve cognitive skills and their patients' physical conditioning. Other day cares serve the broader population and may not be as sensitive to the needs of an Alzheimer's sufferer.

A typical day at an adult day care center can include all the following according to needs and abilities:

- Supervised care
- Activities such as reminiscence, sensory stimulation, music, and art
- Intergenerational activities with visits from children and teens
- Nutritious meals
- Transportation
- Case management
- Recreation and exercise
- Nursing care
- Education
- Family counseling
- Assistance with activities of daily living
- Occupational, speech, and physical therapies

## Facilities for Alzheimer's Care

The types of facilities in the sequence that you may need for your relative include retirement homes with assisted-living programs, licensed residential care homes, dedicated Alzheimer's care facilities, and nursing homes. As mentioned earlier, the Alzheimer's sufferer will go through different stages in which he or she will need different levels of care. The facility you choose must be able to provide that particular level of care needed at that time.

### *Retirement Homes with Assisted Living Programs*

This type of residence will likely have licensed personal care programs that are suited to people with early stage Alzheimer's and symptoms of confusion and short-term memory loss. It may also be the most appropriate choice for a couple where the spouse is independent and taking care of a loved one with early Alzheimer's. CareNeeds assessment will determine whether a residential facility will be safe and appropriate at the outset. As symptoms progress, the residential care facility may not be suitable.

If you and your partner wish to enter a retirement residence, you have to be sure the program is integrated for both independent and assisted living residents.

The accommodations are usually a small apartment where you have all the amenities. You may have a choice of signing up for dining room privileges, and there are usually ongoing group activities.

Some retirement homes have a separate section dedicated to assisted-living residents, but in other residences, there is no segregation. It appears, however, that most retirement residences have some kind of assisted-living programs available, which adds to their appeal to disabled seniors or families trying to place their relative.

### Care Offered

You will have to carefully assess and ask questions about what their care covers. We have all heard the stories of someone being allowed to stay in a facility as long as they are not incontinent, and then having to find another facility. As itemized by the counselor, such as the California Registry, what you are looking for is assistance with bathing and dressing, supervision of medications, assistance with going to the bathroom, management of incontinency care (both bladder and bowel incontinency), and special dietary requirements.

Skilled nursing services are not covered or even allowed to be offered by a retirement residence. If acute or chronic care of a colostomy or necessary injections of medication are required, this has to be prescribed by the resident's doctor and administered by an outside licensed home health agency as needed. Otherwise, the resident would have to immediately be admitted to a nursing home to receive nursing care. Allowing the two systems to intersect, retirement residence and home health care, allows a measure of independence.

### Assisted-Living Facilities

An assisted-living residence combines housing, personalized supportive services, and health care designed to meet the changing needs of people who require help with activities of daily living. Health-care workers who understand wandering behavior and can supervise several people at one time make these facilities an important phase in the sequence of caregiving facilities.

Usually smaller than retirement homes, assisted-living facilities are organized to provide a broad range of services for dependent seniors who can no longer live alone. They are often individual apartments but modified with special adaptations for disabilities. They will have wide doors for wheelchairs, tiled floors, walk-in showers, and emergency call pull cords.

The ALFA describes the following services customarily provided in assisted-living facilities:

- Three meals a day served in a common dining area
- Housekeeping services
- Transportation
- Assistance with eating, bathing, dressing, going to the bathroom, and walking
- Access to health and medical services
- 24-hour security and staff availability
- Emergency call systems for each resident's unit

- Health promotion and exercise programs
- Medication management
- Personal laundry services
- Social and recreational activities

When nuclear families, with a mother and father both working, could no longer afford to have someone at home to take care of parents or grandparents, retirement residences began to gain momentum. With the increase in numbers of seniors and seniors' disabilities, assisted living became another added on feature to retirement homes.

The Assisted Living Federation of America members strive to adhere to the following 10-point philosophy of care:

1. Offering cost-effective quality care that is personalized for individual needs.
2. Fostering independence for each resident.
3. Treating each resident with dignity and respect.
4. Promoting the individuality of each resident.
5. Allowing each resident choice of care and lifestyle.
6. Protecting each resident's right to privacy.

7. Nurturing the spirit of each resident.
8. Involving family and friends, as appropriate, in care planning and implementation.
9. Providing a safe residential environment.
10. Making the assisted-living residence a valuable community asset.

### Costs and Who Pays for Assisted Living?

The cost of assisted living, according to the ALFA, naturally varies with the residence, room size, and the types of services needed by the residents. The range across the nation, however, is from $450 to $6,000 per month. Residents usually pay the cost of assisted living from pensions, insurance, social security, or from family support. Some residences have their own financial assistance programs.

Be warned, government assistance for this type of care has been limited. Some state and local governments offer subsidies for rent or services for low-income elders in the community that they obtain from various sources.

## *Licensed Residential Care Home*

This is a type of assisted-living facility that offers care for moderate to severe stages of Alzheimer's. They are in a home setting, usually have a maximum of six residents, and provide round-the-clock care. For example, in California, there are over 5,100 licensed residential care facilities for the elderly. Residential care is defined as a nonmedical service by caretakers in either a single family residence, retirement residence, or nursing home. Most residential care, more than 90 percent in California, is in single-family dwellings.

Since Alzheimer's is not a disease with physical disabilities per se, skilled caregivers meet most needs, and patients don't require nursing assistance. The only drawback might be for those people who require more activities and stimulation. This can be overcome, however, by linking with community resources that have adult day care programs.

The costs of residential care run about half that of nursing home care. In California, the range is from $850 to $4,000 a month, with an average cost of $1,500 to $1,900, depending on the amount of care needed, the size and quality of the accommodations, and the location of the facility. Few smaller homes will accept Supplemental Security Income (SSI), and if they do, they will require an additional several hundred dollars a month on top. Larger facilities may accept SSI, but only if the resident does not require full-time care.

**How are residential care facilities different from retirement homes?**

As with retirement homes, they are not permitted to provide skilled nursing services, but they provide all other caregiving assistance including help with bathing, dressing, going to the bathroom, and urinary or bowel incontinency care.

## Alzheimer's Dedicated Care Facility

Because of the growing need for Alzheimer's care, more Alzheimer's facilities are opening.

Because they are few at present, the cost for care appears higher than other facilities. This type of facility, which specializes in dementia care, may be what is required for someone in the severe stage of Alzheimer's with aggressive behavior. These facilities are not nursing homes, but rather are licensed as residential care facilities. They are much larger than residential homes with an average of sixty residents. Staff in these facilities have more experience in working with dementia patients.

### Nursing Homes

The final resting place, when your loved one is bedridden, may in fact be back at home. Their care is still challenging but perhaps less so than the wandering and aggressive or dangerous behavior. Otherwise, the final stop for many Alzheimer's patients is a nursing home. The most appropriate facility for someone with advanced and terminal stages of the disease would be a nursing home with a dedicated Alzheimer's care program.

## Hospice Care

A hospice is an end-of-life compassionate care service for people who are terminally ill. It is most often a small residential facility where treatment focuses on well-being rather than a cure. Medications are given for pain management and symptom relief. Hospice services, however, can be provided in the patient's home, in a hospital, in a nursing home, in an assisted-living facility, or wherever the patient resides.

> The goal of hospice is to keep the patient with Alzheimer's as comfortable as possible in the final stages of disease and to provide emotional and spiritual support to the dying relative and his or her family.

The hospice team may include a medical director, the patient's attending physician, nurses, social workers, counselors, clergy, and home health aides. Regular team meetings ensure the best care is given to each patient. A member of the team is usually always on call to family members.

By definition, hospice services are only for people who are terminally ill. To be accepted into hospice care, the following criteria should be met:

- A doctor's diagnosis of end stage Alzheimer's with six months or less to live must be presented.
- The family must consent to hospice services.
- The family must provide a health care proxy or living will signed by the person with Alzheimer's.
- If no proxy or living will is available, the family must provide clear, convincing evidence that the wishes of the person with Alzheimer's are known regarding extraordinary treatment such as resuscitation or tube feeding.

### National Hospice Foundation

The National Hospice Foundation, founded in 1978, changed its name to the National Hospice and Palliative Care Organization (NHPCO) in 2000. NHPCO is the largest nonprofit membership organization in the United States and represents hospice and palliative care programs and professionals in the United States. Its commitment is to improve end-of-life care and expand hospice services to enhance the quality of life for people dying in America. Palliative care was defined in 1990 by the World Health Organization as addressing not just physical pain but also emotional, spiritual, and social pain.

Its headquarters are near Washington, D.C., in Alexandria, Virginia, where it advocates for the terminally ill and their families. For its membership, it develops public and professional educational programs and materials to enhance understanding and availability of hospice and palliative care. NHPCO hosts meetings and seminars on hospice issues, provides technical informational resources to its membership, conducts research, monitors Congressional and regulatory activities, and works closely with other organizations that share an interest in end-of-life care.

NHPCO represents 80 percent of hospices nationwide. According to its statistics, NHPCO estimates that more than 90 percent of the 885,000 hospice patients in 2002 were cared for by its members. More than seven million patients have been served by hospice since 1992. NHPCO helps family members of terminally ill patients locate either in-hospital care or home hospice care. Their toll-free number is S800-658-8898, or you can visit their Web site at *www.hospiceinfo.org*.

## The Hospice Foundation of America

The Hospice Foundation of America is a not-for-profit organization that provides leadership in the development and application of hospice and its philosophy of care. It was chartered in 1982 to help provide fundraising assistance to needy hospices operating in South Florida. This was prior to passage of the Medicare hospice benefit.

In 1990, the Foundation grew to a national level in order to provide leadership and advocate health care for the entire spectrum of end-of-life issues. The Foundation offers professional development, research, public education, and information to assist those who cope either personally or professionally with terminal illness, death, and the process of grief. It offers information on locating a hospice, what questions to ask when interviewing for a hospice, and resources related to hospice care and grieving. The Hospice Foundation of America is supported by contributions from individuals and corporations, grants from foundations, and gifts from associations and civic and fraternal groups.

*Chapter 10*

# Community, State, and National Support

A vast array of support
structures have been erected
in America to help keep the
caregivers healthy and support
them in their task. Caregiving is
very difficult in the beginning
and the difficulty increases as
the disease progresses, so it's
important to know where you
can turn for financial assistance,
reassurance, support groups,
literature, and practical
strategies for coping.

## Small Beginnings

In 1979, a national Alzheimer's association was formed. The new organization, the Alzheimer's Association, was spearheaded by a number of people who had formed Alzheimer's support services in their communities. Those simple beginnings have resulted in Alzheimer's groups and organizations that span the globe.

### Alzheimer's Disease International

Formed in 1984, Alzheimer's Disease International (ADI) is a federation of over sixty-six national Alzheimer's associations around the world. Their role is to help create and support Alzheimer's associations, particularly those in developing countries that depend on the aid of the ADI. ADI began in the United States but is now based in the United Kingdom. Among its organizational tasks are an annual international conference, a World Alzheimer's Day, lobbying for research, providing information, and an Alzheimer's University.

## Community Resources Abound

There are dozens of agencies and organizations that are available to Alzheimer's sufferers and their families.

There are government agencies that can direct you to federally funded services and nonprofit associations that provide information on everything from caregiving to financial planning.

It is necessary to reach out to community support groups for help. As you will see, these organizations have been operating for decades, and usually you can just pick up the phone or go online to find help. Beyond helping individuals with Alzheimer's, many of these organizations also lobby local, state, and national government to increase funding for Alzheimer's care and research.

### *Alzheimer's Disease Education and Referral Center*

In 1990, the U.S. Congress created the Alzheimer's Disease Education and Referral

Center (ADEAR). Their mandate is to "compile, archive, and disseminate information concerning Alzheimer's disease" for health professionals, people with Alzheimer's disease and their families, and the public. The NIA conducts and finances health research for seniors and works closely with ADEAR.

**What is the function of ADEAR?**

ADEAR provides information and materials about the search for causes, treatment, cures, and better diagnostic tools for Alzheimer's that are carefully researched and thoroughly reviewed by NIA scientists and health communicators.

It supplies patients, caregivers, and professionals with a large national database where you can access state, regional, and federally funded services available in your community. You can access their Web site at *www.alzheimers.org.*

## *The Alzheimer's Association*

Founded in 1979, the Alzheimer's Association is the foremost Alzheimer's organization in the United States. It has eighty-one chapters throughout the United States. Branching out from the chapters are 180 Regional Centers and forty-eight Points of Service for a total of 309 sites nationwide.

All Alzheimer's Association chapters are able to offer five core programs and services in the surrounding area. The core services include care consultation, information and referral, support groups, education, and Safe Return/Safety Services. Individual chapters also offer programs and services based on specific community needs. These could entail assistance for people with Alzheimer's who live alone, plus outreach to rural and multicultural populations. Some Association chapters provide funding for local researchers. It can be accessed at *www.alz.org*.

## *Safe Return*

Wandering behavior is common in Alzheimer's disease. Safe Return is a national, government-funded program of the Alzheimer's Association. It was developed to assist in the identification and safe return of individuals with Alzheimer's disease and related dementias who wander off and become lost. This is a unique nationwide program that began in 1993.

> Since 1993, nearly 110,000 individuals have registered in Safe Return nationwide and more than 8,000 individuals have been safely returned to their families and caregivers.

The program utilizes identification products and supports a national photo database and a twenty-four-hour, toll-free emergency crisis line, and offers wandering behavior education and training. Information regarding Safe Return can be found on the Alzheimer's Association Web site.

## *The American Health Assistance Foundation*

The American Health Assistance Foundation (AHAF) is a nonprofit, charitable organization founded in 1973. For over thirty years, this organization has funded research on age-related and degenerative diseases and educated the public about these diseases. AHAF has awarded more than $55 million in grants to sponsor medical research, provides cash grants up to $500 to needy caregivers through its Alzheimer's Family Relief Program, and has given more than $1.9 million in emergency financial assistance to families in need in forty-nine states. Its community outreach works with community organizations to distribute information and educational material, making its presence known by exhibiting at national conferences and meetings and sponsoring conferences on Alzheimer's.

AHAF also provides a variety of published materials about Alzheimer's disease for patients and family caregivers. It has a national toll-free line that provides information, support, and referrals (1-800-437-AHAF, 9 A.M. to 5 P.M. Eastern Standard Time, Monday to Friday).

## *The American Health Care Association*

The American Health Care Association (AHCA) has been in operation since the 1940s. It is a nonprofit federation of affiliated state health organizations, which together represent nearly 12,000 nonprofit and for-profit assisted living, nursing facility, developmentally disabled, and subacute care providers. In total, they care for more than 1.5 million elderly and disabled individuals nationally.

AHCA is the main representative of the long-term care community for the United States and promotes ongoing improvement in the field. AHCA provides information to caregivers on how to choose such a facility and how to pay for it. From its Washington, D.C. headquarters, the association maintains staff working on legislative, regulatory, and public affairs, as well as member services working both internally and externally to assist the interests of government, the general public, and member providers. You can access their Web site at *www.ahca.org*.

The AHCA's established tenets are:

- To improve the standards of service and administration of member nursing homes.
- To secure and merit public and official recognition and approval of the work of nursing homes.
- To adopt and promote programs of education, legislation, and better understanding and mutual cooperation.

The AHCA says their "ultimate focus is on providing quality care to the nation's frail, elderly, and disabled, who are served by the long-term care professionals who comprise AHCA's membership. These providers believe that the individuals whom they serve are entitled to a supportive environment in which professional and compassionate care is delivered."

## *The National Association of Area Agencies on Aging*

The National Association of Area Agencies on Aging (N4A) is the umbrella organization for 655 state Area Agencies on Aging (AAAs) and more than 230 Native American aging programs in the United States. N4A is located in Washington, D.C., where it is a strong advocate for necessary resources for its local aging agencies. The fundamental mission of the AAAs' programs is to help older individuals to remain in their homes and maintain their independence and dignity.

> Local AAAs coordinate and support a wide range of home- and community-based services. Each state has a government Agency on Aging office located in the state capital. The state agency will connect individuals with the nearest local agency in their community.

Referrals include meal delivery, home health workers, transportation services, and caregiver support groups.

N4A operates the Eldercare Locator, a toll-free, nationwide telephone service offering information and referrals for many helpful services for older people in their communities. These include adult day care, respite for caregivers, transportation, home health care, meals on wheels, assistance with housing, and other services available locally. You can access their

Web site at *www.aoa.dhhs.gov*. This service is supported by a cooperative agreement with the U.S. Administration on Aging.

## Government Information

There are many government resources available to seniors. Some of them overlap with other services, and some of them are difficult to find without guidance. Besides providing direct services, various government branches support Alzheimer's organizations and foundations and direct funds to Alzheimer's medical research.

### Resource Directory for Older People

This is a free directory accessed through a toll-free number (1-800-222-2225) coordinated by the National Institute of Aging and the Administration on Aging. The directory is designed to help older people and their families locate national organizations offering health information, legal aid, self-help programs, educational opportunities, social services, consumer advice, or other assistance.

The directory lists over 200 federal agencies, professional societies, private groups, and voluntary programs and provides information to health and legal professionals, social service providers, librarians, and researchers, as well as older people and their families.

It lists federal agencies, Administration on Aging resource centers, professional societies, private groups, and volunteer programs. Some of the organizations listed deal mainly with older people and their families, while others serve professionals who work with older adults, and still others target people of all ages.

### HealthFinder

HealthFinder is a government Web site providing health care information for all ages and includes access to online journals, libraries, an encyclopedia, and medical dictionaries. Specifically for seniors, there is the pension search directory. The site can be accessed at *www .healthfinder.gov*. It has a health library covering prevention and wellness, diseases and conditions, and alternative medicine.

Under the heading, "health care," it provides information about doctors, dentists, public clinics, hospitals, long-term care, nursing homes, health insurance, prescriptions, health fraud, Medicare, Medicaid, and medical privacy. It provides a directory of HealthFinder organizations and health information, as well as Web sites from government agencies, clearinghouses, nonprofits, and universities.

### The National Family Caregivers Association

The National Family Caregivers Association (NFCA) is a grass roots organization of caregivers "created to educate, support, empower, and speak up for the millions of Americans who care for chronically ill, aged, or disabled loved ones." It states that it is "the only constituency organization that reaches across the boundaries of different diagnoses, different relationships and different life stages to address the common needs and concerns of all family caregivers." NFCA is funded by pharmaceutical corporations, health care corporations, and charitable foundations.

One NFCA project is dissemination of the IDentify Alzheimer's Disease (IDAD) free Resource Kit, which includes important information about how to distinguish Alzheimer's disease warning signs from normal aging, resources for caregivers of loved ones newly diagnosed with this illness, and much more. The kit includes *Alzheimer's Disease: What Everyone Should Know,* an educational video featuring TV personality Linda Dano; *Caregiving: What Everyone Should Know,* a brochure written by Dano; *IDentify Alzheimer's Disease Early,* an educational brochure; *Detecting Early Stage Alzheimer's Disease,* a questionnaire; and an educational brochure *Improving Caregiver/Doctor Communications.*

## Starting an Alzheimer's Caregiver Support Group

It is possible that in your small town there is, as yet, no Alzheimer's caregiver support group. So why not start one yourself? Alzheimer's Disease International offers a booklet called "Starting a

Self-Help Group" so you won't have to reinvent the wheel. We will summarize it briefly here. The booklet was created by experienced caregivers who work with support or self-help groups around the world.

The purpose of a self-help group is to meet with people who are sharing the same experience that you are and to offer mutual support. In such a group, you don't have to spend a lot of introductory time explaining what you do, how you feel, or what your stresses are. A few key words like wandering or sundowning, and phrases like "my mother is there but not there," speak volumes to those who are in the same position. The purpose of the group is to:

- Share feelings and experiences.
- Learn more about the disease and giving care.
- Give caregivers an opportunity to talk through problems they are facing or choices they have to make.
- Listen to others who share similar feelings and experiences.
- Help others through the sharing of ideas and information and providing support.

- Gain satisfaction from sharing with and helping others.
- Offer caregivers a break and a chance to get out of the house.
- Encourage and give permission for caregivers to take care of themselves in order to safeguard their health and well-being.
- Remind caregivers that they are not alone.

**Can you cope with the additional demands of organizing a support group?**

You must acknowledge for yourself before embarking on this new project whether you have the time and energy for it.

### Support Group Details

If you want to create a larger group and offer it to other caregivers who need support, then you will need to create a "to do" list. For example, new people will want to know the aim of the group, such as meeting for mutual support, to share feelings and experiences, or to learn more about Alzheimer's and caregiving.

Will you announce your meetings in doctors' offices, at church, in the local newspaper, or as a community event on the radio or local TV? This immediately brings up the question of how many people you can accommodate. You may need to find a large place—a church hall or local community center, or a room at your local library.

Meetings can be weekly, bimonthly, or monthly; it's the group's decision. But the meeting dates and times should be on a set schedule. The group also needs to decide if the meetings are for support or information or both. Will you invite speakers to share information? By information, this doesn't mean just didactic statistics on Alzheimer's; you can also invite psychologists and social workers who can teach coping skills and behavior modification skills.

### Group Dynamics

One or two group leaders are essential for good group dynamics. If you started the group, it doesn't mean you necessarily want to be or should be the group leader. Group leaders must first have the time to coordinate and organize the group; he or she should be a good speaker and be able to make everyone feel that they belong without judging. But don't forget that group leaders are also caregivers and need support, too.

Group rules should be set up early on. These rules are basic to all support groups and help establish a trusting environment:

- All information about members and discussions within the group is kept confidential.
- Members of the group listen and support each other without criticizing or making judgments.
- No one is expected to be the "perfect" caregiver.
- Each member is respected, and all are made to feel equal in the group.
- Each member has a chance to speak if he or she wishes.
- Each member's situation is respected. What is right for one person may not be right for another.

### *How to Run a Meeting*

The duration of the meeting should be set and then the group leader will give each item on the agenda specific times. The group leader greets everyone, welcomes new members, and states the purpose of the group. The rules of the group, including confidentiality, are spoken, especially if there are new members.

Each meeting can have a topic as the focal point of the discussion. It could be about finding caregiver support; medical, financial, or legal problems; or about the larger experience of dealing with Alzheimer's. The group leader opens the discussion and guides it to make sure everyone has an opportunity to speak. At the end of the meeting, the group leader can ask for people to share their thoughts about the meeting and then give a summary of the discussion points. The date and time of the next meeting are announced and the meeting is adjourned. Most groups will have a time for refreshments and mingling at the end of the meeting.

*Chapter 11*

# Insurance, Financial, and Legal Issues

These are tough subjects to write about and tough subjects to read about, especially if you don't have insurance, have limited finances, and can't afford to ask a lawyer for legal advice. It's by focusing on these issues, however, that the real planning for Alzheimer's care takes place. When you know what your resources are, then you can make decisions.

## Types of Insurance

You may have private health insurance that covers all your needs. If not, and you decide to add insurance or change your insurance, make sure you don't have to wait for coverage to be effective.

> You must have a person knowledgeable about insurance review your health insurance very carefully to make sure Alzheimer's is covered and to find any possible loopholes in coverage.

If you have no insurance, there are several government plans in place but you may need some help finding it.

### Employee Benefits

Many workers underutilize their health coverage because they do not read the details of their coverage. Your policy may entitle you to sick leave with pay or short-term disability benefits. Pension plans usually pay full benefits for a disabled worker even before retirement age.

## *COBRA Coverage*

A federal law protects workers' health insurance if they are diagnosed with a condition like Alzheimer's and have to either leave work or cut back on work. It is called the Consolidated Omnibus Budget Reconciliation Act of 1985 (COBRA). It allows you to keep your employer group health care coverage if you have to stop work or cut back to a part-time position.

You must apply for COBRA within sixty days of change in job status. And it may be extended up to three years. The only drawback is that you must pay the full premium. COBRA provides stopgap insurance until you find other coverage or are accepted for Medicare.

## *Disability Insurance*

This can be a private or a work-related policy. Most policies are sold on the basis of providing you with between 60 and 70 percent of your income. If it is a private policy, you may have opted to pay for a higher amount. Employer-driven policies are tax deductible. Personal disability policies are tax-free.

## Medicare

Medicare is a federal health insurance program that provides coverage for people age sixty-five or older who are also receiving social security retirement benefits. You have to have paid into the social security system for ten years to be eligible. Some people under age sixty-five who have disabilities and people with permanent kidney failure on dialysis or awaiting kidney transplant are also accepted.

### Medicare: Part A and Part B

There are two parts to Medicare. The first, called Part A, covers hospitalization, nursing, hospice, and some home health care. Part A is an automatic free benefit at age sixty-five to individuals if they or their spouse paid Medicare taxes while they worked. Those who did not pay

Medicare taxes while working may be able to purchase Part A coverage.

Part B is medical insurance that covers medically necessary doctors' services, outpatient hospital care, some specialty services such as physical and occupational therapists, and some home health care. Part B can be purchased. The rate changes yearly.

## *What Does Medicare Cover?*

According to the Fisher Center for Alzheimer's Research Foundation at the Rockefeller University, Medicare covers 80 percent of certain medical services for the treatment of Alzheimer's disease.

The Alzheimer's services Medicare now covers include "reasonable and necessary" doctors' visits; physical, occupational, or speech therapy; psychotherapy or behavioral management therapy by a mental health professional; and skilled homecare services.

A gap in Medicare was filled in November 2003 when a new Medicare drug law came into effect. Medicare will now cover prescription drugs.

### Medicare Health Plans

There are three different ways to receive Medicare benefits. The first is the Original Medicare Plan. Because this plan doesn't cover all eventualities in a health crisis, however, you may need to add Medigap, which supplements Medicare. Or your former employer could still be providing supplemental coverage.

The other two plans, which add on to the original Medicare Plan, are sold by private companies. They are called Medicare Plus Choice plans and include Medicare Managed Care Plan and Medicare Private Fee-for-Service plans. Medicare Managed Care is a Medicare HMO, or health maintenance organization. It may provide the additional benefit of prescription medication coverage, but it usually restricts access to its own list of doctors and hospitals.

Private Fee-for-Service plans are called Medicare + Choice health plans. They are offered by private insurance companies, which are under contract to the Medicare program. Medicare pays the Private Fee-for-Service organization an agreed upon amount of money every month to arrange for the extended health care coverage for Medicare beneficiaries who have enrolled in these plans.

These plans entitle beneficiaries to go to any eligible doctor or hospital anywhere in the United States that is willing to provide care and accepts the member's Private Fee-for-Service plans' terms of payment.

### Medicaid

Medicaid is a government program run jointly by local, state, and federal agencies and administered by each individual state's welfare agency for people with limited incomes and little or no assets. Criteria for eligibility and benefits vary from state to state, but it can be used by people who have exhausted their own resources. Medicaid covers all or a portion of nursing home costs, and that's where most of Medicaid dollars are spent. Some states, however, are developing home care and community care options. A person with Alzheimer's can qualify for long-term care under Medicaid only if he or she has minimal income and cash assets. Such people will also be covered for hospice care if not covered by Medicare.

## Financial Issues and Alzheimer's

A diagnosis of Alzheimer's comes with the crushing reality that you might not be able to continue working for many more years. Immediately, your thoughts spiral out to concerns about how you can afford your future care. You wonder how expensive Alzheimer's care is and how long you will live with the disease. And will you have to depend on your family for financial support? These are very scary issues, but when you start talking about them with your family and friends and find support networks, you will be able to make financial plans for the future.

You may have disability insurance that gives you some regular income. You may have planned for retirement and have income either through your workplace or through individual retirement accounts (IRAs), annuities, investment assets (stocks and bonds, savings accounts, real estate, etc.), and personal property (jewelry and artwork). If you own your home, money from the sale of your home can be invested, or a new mortgage can be taken out on your home. If your assets are limited, financial resources are available through government assistance or community-based organizations.

### Who can help you plan your financial future?

Your banker, the person handling your retirement savings, or a financial planner along with a knowledgeable family member or friend, can help to create a financial picture of your future.

With their support, you will need to look at the following health-care expenses: ongoing doctor visits, prescription medications, home care services, and possible future nursing home care. You will also need to decide who will manage your finances when you no longer can.

## *A Financial Advisor*

Once you and a family member have tackled the financial paperwork, it's time to sit down with a financial professional who works in eldercare. A financial planner, estate planner, or your banker will have information about financial support for people with Alzheimer's. Your banker will also be able to advise about direct bill payment and direct deposit of incoming money including your social security checks.

## *Financing Long-Term Housing*

The mostly costly aspect of Alzheimer's will be your future housing. After the family or support system can no longer provide the necessary care, it's a matter of finding out about the expense of residential care and nursing home care and planning appropriately.

A knowledgeable financial consultant will advise you on what to do about family assets. If titles are transferred or wealth given to family members, you may not be entitled to Medicaid if you need it in the future. One rule is that anything you give away up to three years before applying to Medicaid is still part of your income. These legal issues, and also tax issues, need to be investigated before making any decisions.

### Tax Deductions and Alzheimer's

Long-term care costs may all be deductible medical expenses. And they may also be deductible on another family member's tax return. The criteria are that the deductible medical expenses must total more than 7.5 percent of adjusted gross income.

### Federal Assistance

The National Council on Aging provides a service called Benefits Checkup that matches the financial statistics of an elderly person with available state and federal assistance programs. Benefits Checkup responds to thousands of requests every day to find programs for people over the age of fifty-five that may pay for some of their costs of prescription drugs, health care, utilities, and other essential items or services.

Benefits Checkup is linked to over 1,100 federal, state, local, and private programs. They include: prescription assistance, health care programs, nutrition programs, property tax programs, veteran's assistance, housing assistance, and financial assistance. Their Web site is located at *www.benefitscheckup.org.*

## Legal Issues and Alzheimer's

While organizing your financial paperwork, you will also want to put your legal paperwork in order. Legal papers include your will and a living will and directives on how you want your care to evolve.

Elder law is a growing field, and you will want to choose a lawyer who is familiar with issues related to Alzheimer's. The family member who is helping you sort out your financial and legal affairs should be present at any meetings with your lawyer. If you can't afford an attorney, you can obtain free legal advice through your local

Legal Aid Society, Area Agency on Aging, or nonprofit legal assistance organizations.

## *Planning for the Future*

Planning for care begins to evolve once you start gathering insurance, financial, and legal papers. Legal and financial planning should begin as soon as possible after a diagnosis has been made. Exploring care options early will give you the comfort and security of knowing what lies ahead in terms of health care and living arrangements.

According to Joseph Jackson of ElderCare Advisors, Inc., because Alzheimer's is becoming the most disabling chronic illness in the United States, it is putting an incredible strain on all available social services. This means people with Alzheimer's and their caregivers will need to be much more resourceful in their planning for Alzheimer's care. Jackson outlines a new practice model for planning care called Community LifeCare Planning (CLCP) and four basic steps in the Alzheimer's CarePlan.

1. Advance Directives
2. Estate Inventory
3. CareNeeds Assessment
4. Defining the Options

### Advance Directives

Advance directives are legally binding documents that allow you to state your preferences regarding ongoing and future treatment and care. Jackson says that being able to execute advance directives is one of the best arguments for early diagnosis. Taking the time to create your advance directives allows you to make your own decision about how you want your care to evolve and who will be in charge of your care and your finances.

Jackson describes five advance directives:

1. A power of attorney
2. A health care proxy
3. A will
4. A living will
5. A Do Not Resuscitate (DNR) order

### *Power of Attorney*

A power of attorney is a document in which you empower someone to legally act on your behalf whose actions are deemed to be your actions. You will need to appoint such a person who will be called your agent. This will usually be a trusted family member or friend. It's best, however, if the whole family agrees who this person will be to prevent rifts in the future.

The term durable power of attorney means that your agent can continue to act on your behalf when you are no longer able to make decisions for yourself.

This is very important in Alzheimer's because you don't want your resources to be cut off if no one is there to sign the checks or deposit your income. A durable power of attorney for health care will allow your agent to make all decisions regarding your health.

In order to make a power of attorney durable, it must be stated in the terms that the power of attorney remains in effect when you become incapacitated.

### Health Care Proxy

Someone who makes health care decisions for you when you are unable is called a health care proxy. It is someone you legally appoint to perform this service when you are still competent and is usually a family member. There is a standard health care proxy form signed in front of two witnesses where you designate your choice and also note specific health care choices you would like them to make for you. For example, if you do not wish to have any surgery, intravenous feedings, a respirator, or CPR, you can note that choice. If you didn't have a health proxy, your doctor may be obliged to give you medical and surgical treatments that you would have rejected if you were able to. The health care proxy only comes into effect when your doctor finds that you are no longer able to make decisions.

### Wills and the Do Not Resuscitate Order

A will is a document you create that names an executor to manage your estate after you die, and also names beneficiaries that will share your estate according to your wishes. The executor is usually known before the will is read after your death and is often the same person who helps you manage your ongoing finances.

A living will is a more formal advance directive that states your preferences for future medical care decisions, especially the use of artificial life support systems. If it is your decision not to be put on life supports, you have the legal right to limit or forgo other medical efforts.

A Do Not Resuscitate directive states that you do not want "heroic measures" taken to save your life in the event of a heart attack or stroke. Copies of these documents can go to your doctor, lawyer, family, and caregiver.

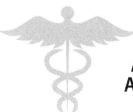

*Appendix A*

# Alzheimer's Associations

**Alzheimer's Association**

800-272-3900

*www.alz.org*

**Alzheimer's Disease Education and Referral Center (ADEAR)**

800-438-4380

*www.alzheimer's.org/adear*

**American Association of Retired Persons (AARP)**

202-434-2277

*www.aarp.org*

**American Health Assistance Foundation (AHAF)**

800-437-2423

*www.ahaf.org*

**American Health Care Association (AHCA)**

800-555-9414

*www.ahca.org*

**Area Agencies on Aging**

Check your local phone book under "Aging" in the State Government pages

**Benefits CheckUp**

The National Council on Aging

*www.benefitscheckup.org*

**Eldercare Locator**

800-677-1116

*www.aoa.dhhs.gov*

**FamilyCareAmerica**

*www.familycareamerica.com*

**HealthFinder**

*www.healthfinder.gov*

**Medicare**

800-772-1213

*www.medicare.gov*

**National Hospice and Palliative Care Organization**

800-658-8898

*www.nhpco.org*

**National Institute on Aging**

800-222-2225

*www.nih.gov*

**Social Security Information Hotline**

800-772-1213

*www.ssa.gov*

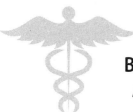

*Appendix B*

# Books about
# Alzheimer's

Bell, Virginia, and David Troxel. *The Best Friends Approach to Alzheimer's Care*. (Health Professions Press, 2003).

Berman, Claire. *Caring for Yourself While Caring for Your Aging Parents: How to Help, How to Survive*. (Owl Books, 2001).

Brackey, Jolene. *Creating Moments of Joy for the Person with Alzheimer's or Dementia: A Journal for Caregivers*. (Purdue University Press, 2000).

Castleman, Michael, et al. *There's Still a Person in There: The Complete Guide to Treating and Coping with Alzheimer's*. (Perigee, 2000).

Coste, Joanne Koenig. *Learning to Speak Alzheimer's: A Groundbreaking Approach for Everyone Dealing with the Disease*. (Houghton Mifflin Company, 2003).

DeBaggio, Thomas. *Losing My Mind: An Intimate Look at Life with Alzheimer's*. (Free Press, 2002).

Dowling, James R. *Keeping Busy: A Handbook of Activities for Persons with Dementia*. (Johns Hopkins University Press, 1995).

Fitzray, B. J. *Alzheimer's Activities: Hundreds of Activities for Men and Women with Alzheimer's Disease and Related Disorders.* (Rayve Productions, 2001).

Kuhn, Daniel, and David A. Bennett. *Alzheimer's Early Stages: First Steps for Family, Friends, and Caregivers.* (Hunter House, 2003).

Loverde, Joy. *The Complete Eldercare Planner, Second Edition: Where to Start, Which Questions to Ask, and How to Find Help.* (Three Rivers Press, 2000).

Mace, Nancy L., and Peter V. Rabins. *The 36-Hour Day: A Family Guide to Caring for Persons with Alzheimer's Disease, Related Dementing Illnesses, and Memory Loss in Later Life.* (Warner Books, 2001).

Marcell, Jacqueline. *Elder Rage, or Take My Father . . . Please!: How to Survive Caring for Aging Parents.* (Impressive Press, 2001).

Petersen, Ronald C., M.D. (Editor) *Mayo Clinic on Alzheimer's Disease.* (Mayo Clinic, Kensington Publishing Corporation, 2002).

Shenk, David. *The Forgetting: Alzheimer's: Portrait of an Epidemic.* (Anchor Books, 2003).

Sheridan, Carmel. *Failure Free Activities for the Alzheimer's Patient.* (Elder Books, 1997).

Strauss, Claudia J. *Talking to Alzheimer's: Simple Ways to Connect When You Visit with a Family Member or Friend.* (New Harbinger Publications, 2001).

*Appendix C*

# Questions to Ask
# the Nursing Home

- *Does staff respond quickly to requests for assistance?*

- *Are residents involved in a variety of activities?*

- *What are the base costs? What are the add-on costs (e.g., laundry, bandages, beauty salon)?*

- *Is the facility Medicare or Medicaid certified?*

- *How will the staff monitor your loved one's care?*

- *Is there an adequate staff-to-resident ratio?*

- *Is privacy respected?*

- *Is there a qualified social worker on staff?*

- *Does the home have contact with community groups such as pet therapy programs and Scouts?*

- *Does the resident or family participate in developing the care plan?*

- *Is there fresh water at bedside?*

- *How many residents share a bathroom? Do bathrooms have hand grips or rails near all toilet and bathing areas? Is there a call button inside?*

- *Who plans the meals? How are special dietary needs met?*

- *What arrangements are made for honoring religious preferences?*

- *Is there a family council for residents? When does it meet and who coordinates it?*

- *Is there a physician available for emergencies?*

- *What is the billing procedure? Will you be informed of any changes?*

- *How is personal laundry handled? Will you need to do it yourself?*

- *Is there a system to protect wanderers?*

# Index